# New Thinking about Mental Health and Employment

Edited by

**Bob Grove** PhD

**Jenny Secker** PhD

**Patience Seebohm** MA

Foreword by

**Robert E Drake**

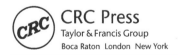

**CRC Press**
Taylor & Francis Group
Boca Raton  London  New York

CRC Press is an imprint of the
Taylor & Francis Group, an **informa** business

**Radcliffe Publishing Ltd**
18 Marcham Road
Abingdon
Oxon OX14 1AA
United Kingdom

**www.radcliffe-oxford.com**
Electronic catalogue and worldwide online ordering facility

---

British Library Cataloguing in Publication Data

A catalogue record for this book is available from the British Library

ISBN: 1 85775 667 3

Typeset by Action Publishing Technology Ltd, Gloucester

# Contents

# Foreword

I have yet to meet an individual with severe mental health problems whose life goal is to be a stable but chronically disabled patient. Yet this is precisely how mental healthcare systems have been constructed – as though the goal were to help people adjust to a life dominated by illness, inactivity and segregation from mainstream society! This unwanted outcome is what disability advocates refer to derisively as the 'disability gulag'.

People with long-term health problems and disabilities have of course the same life goals as the rest of us – to participate in personally meaningful social, educational, vocational and other community activities. People want to be productive, to earn money, to contribute and participate in their communities. It should be no surprise that people with long-term mental health problems express vocational goals in the UK, the US, the Netherlands, Canada, Hong Kong, Australia, and every other place where they have been asked.

As Bob Grove, Jenny Secker and Patience Seebohm make clear in this delightful book, the service technology for helping people with mental health problems achieve their vocational goals has been rapidly developing for at least 20 years.

One major impediment to achieving a consensus on meaningful employment as the goal of the mental health system has been a lack of clear and consistent voice. Narrow books and journal articles on mental illness, disability, health services, rehabilitation, or recovery offer limited and, in many ways limiting, views. One often hears researchers emphasising 'broken brain' paradigms, advocates calling for 'recovery' paradigms, insurers asking for 'cost-effective' models, and policy makers asking for a modicum of consistency in definitions, services and goals. Legislators wonder why these tribes do not talk with one another and sometimes seem content to create a self-destructive din.

Synthesis of voice is precisely the remarkable contribution of this book. Edited books rarely achieve coherence, consistency and quality. But this volume beautifully brings together the perspectives of service users, advocates, professionals, researchers and policy makers. The message should be clear to all. Effective services can and should enable those with serious mental health problems and disabilities to return to functional and meaningful vocational roles: this is a fundamental goal that is eminently attainable.

If I might be permitted to go one step further, I also anticipate that the current technology of supported employment will continue to improve substantially in the near future. New approaches will enable us to overcome more completely societal barriers, service system problems and individual difficulties. Employment outcomes will continue to improve, and I for one hope that Bob

Grove, Jenny Secker, Patience Seebohm and the other contributors to this book will continue to work their magic.

Robert E Drake, MD, PhD
Professor and Director of Research
Dartmouth Medical School
Lebanon, New Hampshire
USA
*April 2005*

# About the editors

**Bob Grove** joined the Sainsbury Centre for Mental Health in 2003 to lead the Employment Programme, which advises government and local authorities on policy implementation. His recent work includes writing employment guidance on the implementation of the government's Learning Disability Strategy and the National Service Framework for Mental Health, both commissioned by the Department of Health. He is currently on secondment to the Department of Health, working on the incapacity benefit reform pilots. He has written widely on disability and employment issues.

**Jenny Secker** is Professor of Mental Health with Anglia Polytechnic University and the South Essex Partnership NHS Trust. She qualified as a mental health nurse in 1979 and as a social worker in 1984. Since completing her PhD at Edinburgh University in 1991, she has pursued a career in health and social care research, focusing on mental health. Before taking up her current post, Jenny was Senior Research Fellow at the Institute for Applied Health and Social Policy, King's College London, where she worked with Bob Grove and Patience Seebohm on several major programmes of research and service development aimed at improving mental health service users' chances of finding and keeping a job. Her research interests continue to centre on mental health and social exclusion.

**Patience Seebohm** has worked with the Employment Programme led by Bob Grove since 1998, first at the Institute for Applied Health and Social Policy, King's College London, and now at the Sainsbury Centre for Mental Health. Her work focused first on increasing paid employment for people supported by community mental health teams (Care Programme to Work), then explored user-led support in employment (Unlocking Potential). Now, much of her work is concerned with increasing paid employment for people with mental health problems from black and minority ethnic communities, including the production of a video, *Better Must Come*, in partnership with Mellow, East London.

# About the contributors

**Graham Cockshutt** is coordinator of the User Support and Employment Service in Sheffield, which promotes and supports the employment aspirations of mental health service users. He also coordinates the Unlocking Potential Project (funded by the Department of Health), a service user run and led support network for people returning, or looking to return, to employment. He was co-founder of the Sheffield Hearing Voices Group and in 2003 received the Outstanding Achiever of the Year award in the NHS/Social Services Yorkshire Workforce Awards. Graham participates in and presents training sessions with students and workers in both voluntary and statutory agencies locally and nationally, working regularly with JobCentre Plus staff to raise awareness of mental health issues.

**Paul Grey** describes himself as someone who has overcome not only the mental health systems but also the 'system', against the odds. He is a multi-gifted motivational and inspirational speaker and writer and an experienced consultant. Paul is now married with a three-year-old son. His business, Grey Services, aims to develop social firms and offer real employment. He is also an associate consultant with the Sainsbury Centre for Mental Health, where he is facilitating the establishment of a national black mental health user network called Inspire and Influence (I&I). His purpose in life is to inspire, encourage and educate.

**Mo Hutchison** has a degree in psychology and has worked for a local Mind group as a day centre coordinator and for regional Mind as a project manager, based in Kent. She became a user consultant in 1996, working mainly for the then Centre for Mental Health Services Development to which she was appointed Senior User Consultant in 1998, remaining in the post until July 2003. She has undertaken freelance work as a user trainer and researcher for a number of organisations including the Department of Health, Mental Health Media and Rethink. She was appointed Project Worker for a safer psychiatric wards initiative in March 2004. She lives in Kent and has three children, three cats and one husband – not necessarily in that order.

**John Marshall** has been Mental Health Employment Co-ordinator for Rethink Graphics in Brentwood, Essex, since 1998. John's experiences as a service user have helped greatly in his positive approach to working with clients. He assists people to explore which skills they enjoy using, whilst considering which areas of employment are of particular interest to them. He believes this positive approach results not only in regained employment but also in employment from which the individual gains genuine satisfaction and the motivation to progress and recover.

**Helen Membrey** is a Service Improvement Manager on a three-year modernisation initiative funded by Guy's and St Thomas' Charitable Foundation. The aim of the programme is to work in partnership with service users and staff across the acute trusts, community services, primary care, social services and other generic services to transform stroke, sexual health and kidney disease services in Lambeth and Southwark. Helen's experience includes a number of social research roles and she spent over two years at the Institute for Applied Health and Social Policy at King's College London, working with Jenny Secker and Bob Grove on a research programme exploring the support and barriers to employment for people who use mental health services. She has an MSc in Social Research and has co-authored a number of publications on the subject of mental health and employment.

**Mary Nettle** became a user of mental health services in 1978 and turned this negative into a positive in 1992 when she became a mental health user consultant. She is involved in presenting the user perspective in all aspects of mental health with a particular interest in user-led research. Current posts held include: honorary fellow of Brunel University; Mental Health Act Local Commissioner; Involve (formerly Consumers in NHS Research) member; lay reviewer and inspector with the Healthcare Commission; Chair of the European Network of Users (ex) Users and Survivors of Psychiatry; and member of the Disabled Women's Committee of the European Disability Forum.

**Rachel Perkins** is both a user and a provider of mental health services. She is a Consultant Clinical Psychologist and Clinical Director of Adult Mental Health Services at South West London and St George's Mental Health NHS Trust, vice-chair of the Manic Depression Fellowship and a member of both the Disability Rights Commission's Mental Health Action Group and the National Social Inclusion Implementation Team. In 1995 she established the Pathfinder User Employment Project, a programme to increase employment opportunities within mental health services for people who have themselves experienced mental health problems.

**Miles Rinaldi** is the Vocational Services Manager for South West London and St George's Mental Health NHS Trust. He also works on a part-time secondment on the implementation of the National Social Inclusion Programme within the National Institute for Mental Health in England (NIMHE). Prior to NIMHE, Miles worked on a part-time secondment on the Mental Health project at the Social Exclusion Unit, Office of the Deputy Prime Minister. He has a BA (Hons) in Music and Philosophy and a Postgraduate Diploma in Psychology. Miles has published research on mental health and employment and the self-management of manic depression.

**Justine Schneider** trained and practised as a social worker before becoming a researcher. She worked freelance before taking up posts first with the Personal

Social Services Research Unit at the University of Kent, then at the University of Durham and most recently at the University of Nottingham, where she now holds a chair in mental health and social care in the Department of Sociology and Social Policy, which is sponsored by Nottinghamshire Healthcare Trust. Her interest in employment stems from a placement as a social work student. Her PhD thesis, *A rationale for employment of people with mental health problems* (1998, University of Kent), was based on research into the costs and benefits of six work schemes. With Jenny Secker, Bob Grove and Mike Floyd, she is currently evaluating supported employment in England in the European Social Fund supported SESAMI project.

**Jo Shenton** currently works part-time at Rethink Graphics in Brentwood, Essex, where she teaches computer training to service users, helps out in the shop, does some design work and helps run the service user meetings. Jo also works part-time as an Indian head massage therapist, takes a sculpture class and keeps an allotment. She has had two solo art exhibitions and plans for another two in the near future. She is also involved with researching into mental health issues with Jenny Secker. Jo lives independently in Brentwood and believes that, considering she used to be so afraid of being alone and couldn't see an end to the long, dark tunnel of depression, this is nothing short of a miracle. She is convinced that if she can do it, so can anyone.

**Tina Thomas** is a psychologist who specialises in employment and mental health, health psychology and adolescent mental health. In 2001, she completed her doctorate in Psychology at Deakin University, Melbourne, Australia, and went on to work at the Institute for Applied Health and Social Policy (IAHSP) at King's College London with Bob Grove and Jenny Secker. During her time at IAHSP, Tina was the primary researcher on a project to evaluate a job retention service for people with mental health problems. Following this, Tina worked on the consultation document for the Social Exclusion Unit, which examined current issues of social exclusion for people with mental health problems. Tina is currently working at Deakin University and practising as a psychologist.

**Richard Watts** was born in London in 1977. He lives in Brentwood, Essex, and is a freelance writer, contributing articles to newsletters and magazines and working on his first novel. He was educated at Reading University, where he studied English. Richard is also a mental health service user, having first suffered mental ill health at the age of 12. He is a seasoned hospital inmate and now writes about his experiences for the benefit of others. Richard is a committed Christian and his hobbies include playing the violin, walking his dog and making people laugh.

# Acknowledgements

The survey data in Chapter 2 were published in Secker J, Grove B, Seebohm P (2001) Challenging barriers to employment, training and education for mental health service users: the service user's perspective. *Journal of Mental Health.* 10(4): 395–404.

The survey described in Chapter 5 was administered by Richard Wistow, Centre for Public Mental Health, University of Durham. The reliability of the supported employment adherence scale was calculated by David Woof, Statistics Consultancy Unit, University of Durham. Sue Sharp and Lisa Naylor of the Department for Work and Pensions kindly checked the accuracy of the information about their provision.

The study described in Chapter 7 was published in Secker J, Membrey H, Grove B *et al.* (2002) Recovering from illness or recovering your life? Implications of clinical versus social models of recovery from mental illness for employment support services. *Disability and Society.* 17(4): 403–18.

The study on which Chapter 8 draws was published in Seebohm P, Secker J (2003) Increasing the vocational focus of the community mental health team. *Journal of Interprofessional Care.* 17(3): 281–91.

Some of the data included in Chapter 15 were published in Rinaldi M, McNeil K, Firn M *et al.* (2004) What are the benefits of evidence-based supported employment for patients with first-episode psychosis? *Psychiatric Bulletin.* 28: 281–4.

Our grateful thanks to all the people who have worked with us over the past few years in exploring new ways of thinking about employment and mental health. Some of you have contributed chapters, others are acknowledged in the text, but it is impossible to acknowledge all those who have been allies in our endeavours. We have learnt a great deal with your help and we hope to continue doing so in the years ahead.

Bob Grove
Jenny Secker
Patience Seebohm
*April 2005*

# Introduction: rethinking employment and mental health

Bob Grove, Jenny Secker and Patience Seebohm

Most people who suffer from periods of mental ill health would like to work and yet less than 20% are in employment. For those with a diagnosis of schizophrenia, the unemployment rate is probably nearer to 95%. People with mental health problems are the least employed of any group of disabled people. The knock-on effects of this are huge, both in personal terms – living on benefits, strains on close relationships, severely restricted social lives – and for the taxpayer in losses to productivity and tax revenues, and in maintaining almost a million adults of working age in economic inactivity.

Why is this? Is there something about mental ill health that makes unemployment inevitable? The common perception would certainly suggest that this is so. 'I have enough problems recruiting and retaining good staff anyway', said one employer who is also the trustee of a large mental health charity. 'Why would I want to employ people who are mentally ill?'

There are a number of assumptions in this statement which are worth unpacking. First, in the employer's mind there is a gulf between his existing workforce – by his own admission hard to recruit, not always up to standard and difficult to hold on to – and a future workforce with people with mental health problems added. This imagined gulf does not stand up to close scrutiny. The employer probably does not know how many people in his current workforce have a history of mental ill health because they are unlikely to have mentioned the fact. Second, there is an assumption that good, reliable, loyal staff could not be found among those who have had a diagnosis of mental illness. Third, there is a clear assumption that if he does employ people who are known to have had mental health problems, his difficulties as an employer will increase. The implications of these assumptions lead to the conclusion that sensible employers will screen out people with a history of mental health problems and therefore the only possible reason for employing them is essentially charitable.

Where do employers get these discriminatory assumptions? Is it from personal experience? Maybe. Just one case of a difficult personnel problem with someone who has shown signs of mental distress will immediately colour the employer's view even if equally difficult situations without a suggestion of mental ill health are regarded as an occasional hazard of running a business.

Is it because of what the employer is or is not told about the individual's condition and the likelihood of recovery? How many GPs have the confidence, skills or time to prescribe a gradual return to work or really communicate with employers, even where they suspect that a patient would be better off going back to work? How many psychiatrists or ward staff routinely ask on admission whether the person has a job and whether they want to try and keep it? Would they know what to say or do if the answer was 'yes'?

In fact, many service users say that their employment needs are not only ignored by mental health professionals but actively discouraged. Some GPs are reported to encourage people to stay off work as long as possible. For people with more severe conditions, it is not unknown for psychiatrists to feel they have to help service users to be 'realistic' by telling them or their relatives they will never work again. Faced with such pessimism among clinicians, is it surprising that employers are wary about recruiting or retaining people once they have the mental patient label?

Of course, the damage is not only to people's chances of employment. Relentless negativity about a person's ability to work or contribute to the life of the community has a corrosive effect on self-confidence and all the internal psychological mechanisms that enable us to feel in control, perform tasks, manage social situations and put up with the vicissitudes of life. The patient role for people with mental health problems can last way beyond the point where the original depression or psychosis is under control or gone away altogether. It says much for the resilience of people who use mental health services that so many retain their employment ambitions through long periods of unemployment and discouragement from those around them.

Is it possible to change this state of affairs or is unemployment an inevitable consequence of mental ill health for most people? The writers of this book believe that there is strong evidence that it is not inevitable, that we can change things for the majority of people if we approach things in the right way and with the right spirit.

This is no small task. It will involve challenging some of our most basic assumptions. We sometimes forget that even the most severe mental distress is comparatively short-lived in its acute forms. Even where the symptoms recur, there are long periods when people are quite able to work and lead fulfilling lives. We have got better and better at keeping people out of hospital. We have, however, made little or no progress in dealing with the most damaging and long-lasting consequences of mental ill health – the journey to social exclusion and disability. We believe there is good evidence that the journey is not directly related to either the nature or severity of a person's mental health problems. Everyone who acquires a diagnosis is at risk but for none is unemployment inevitable. As several of the contributors to this book vividly illustrate, by dint of personal resilience and good fortune in the support they receive, people who need to use mental health services can lead normal employed lives, whatever their diagnosis. If this is possible for some people, why is it not possible for everyone?

We also know that once a person is on the path to exclusion, the longer it goes on the harder it is to get back. However, there is also evidence that the journey can be stopped and reversed. If it is possible to do this then it makes sense both in personal and economic terms to get in early with practical support and assistance. This is particularly important if someone is in employment when they come into contact with services. For most of us, employment is at the centre of our lives – other parts of our lives are contingent on the income and relationships sustained by employment. Allowing someone to lose a job, just because no one has thought to ask if it can be held open, is a reckless waste of a life.

However, we are not just advocating changes to our attitudes and ways of dealing with mental ill health and employment. It is our belief that the implications of what we are saying about helping people with mental health problems to have a working life extend into other life domains. We are talking about recovery in its broadest sense and how we can create the conditions in which it is possible for people to undertake that sometimes hazardous and fearful journey. There has to be both hope and faith in the eventual outcome of the journey, not only in the individual but in the community around them. For all their successes in alleviating distress, mental health services have failed utterly to support the development of faith and hope. This has had massive, long-lasting consequences, especially for people with severe forms of mental distress.

## Old evidence, new thinking about schizophrenia

Schizophrenia is the most frightening, hopeless and stigmatising diagnosis a person can receive. There is evidence to suggest that employment rates for people with schizophrenia are very low indeed and getting worse. However, even with this diagnosis, we believe it is possible and very desirable for most people to be supported in paid work if that is what they want. This is not just a wild dream. In a seminal article, Arnold Kruger fundamentally challenges the view of schizophrenia as an illness from which full recovery is impossible.[1] Calling his article 'Schizophrenia, recovery and hope', he presents his challenge from two distinct points of view: the way the terminology we use is constructed and evidence from long-term studies on recovery from schizophrenia.

The first area of challenge is in the use of diagnostic terminology. Going through all the various Diagnostic and Statistical Manuals of Mental Disorder (DSMs – the US equivalent of the International Classification of Disease used in Europe), Kruger points out that from the beginning until the present day the diagnosis of schizophrenia is associated with progressive mental and social deterioration. Indeed, such deterioration is one of the defining criteria.

Kraepelin, who was the first to identify what he called 'dementia praecox', which means early-onset dementia, said that the only difference between what was later called schizophrenia and manic depressive psychosis is that: 'Manic depressive insanity is characterised by the recurrence of groups of mental symptoms throughout the life of the individual, *not* leading to mental deterioration'.[2]

This, Kruger argues, has from the beginning created a process of negative circular reasoning about schizophrenia. If the condition is apparently chronic and hopeless then it is schizophrenia. If it is schizophrenia it must be chronic and hopeless. He points out that all psychotic states that last less than six months are excluded from the category of schizophrenia. No matter how much they might look like schizophrenia, they are given other names. This 'official litany of hopelessness and doom' arises therefore from the creation of a diagnostic category which has been shaped to exclude people who recover. Kruger adds that, given this, it is unsurprising that suicide is frequently associated with the condition.

Kruger's second line of challenge comes from long-term empirical studies of the course of schizophrenia. Up to the 1950s, long-term follow-up studies had stopped at around 10 years and showed the familiar and predicted process of mental deterioration and chaotic, unhappy lives. However, some very long-term studies lasting 20–30 years have now produced quite startling evidence, indicating that even into the second and third decade of the illness, there is still potential for full or partial recovery. The Vermont Study[3] took as its cohort people placed in tertiary care settings from the back wards, recruited as 'profoundly ill, severely disabled long-stay patients' who met the DSM-1 guidelines for schizophrenia. The study, which followed people for up to four decades, showed that at an average of 32 years after discharge 26% were employed, of whom three-quarters were earning a satisfactory income. Forty-nine per cent were or had been in long-term relationships, 90% lived independently and 68% were suffering only mild symptoms (such as insomnia) and were functioning at a level most people would consider normal. In Europe, a more recent international study following people up after 15 and 25 years has revealed strikingly similar results.[4]

## Towards a good news paradigm

All this adds up in Kruger's view (and ours) to the need for a revolutionary new paradigm, which restores hope and abolishes the artificial and false dichotomy between poor outcome schizophrenia and the other states that differ from it only in the fact that people make a full recovery. Kruger proposes a continuum on which the various schizophrenias exist and construes the condition in its most severe form as a long-term but time-limited condition from which most people make a full recovery.

You might think that this discovery was good news which mental health professionals would have been keen to make widely known. But this seems not to have been the case.

> We've got a completely different perspective on schizophrenia and other psychoses... but the notion of long-term improvement in schizophrenia has triggered tremendous resistance over the years. It's been difficult for us to present this to the world and have it well received. The findings emerging from the Vermont Study in the early 80s startled the daylights out of us.[5]

Given what we know of the ravages and long-term nature of schizophrenia, do these findings really matter? Kruger argues (and our many conversations with service users over the years support his view) that the whole picture of schizophrenia is 'radically changed by the addition of hope'. Essentially, people will find the courage to keep going through the bad times if they know that eventually they will end. This view receives first-hand support from Simon Champ, an Australian service user.

> At this stage I began to see that while I might not be able to control my illness, I could control my attitude to it. I began to see strong links between quality of life and the attitude one had to illness. I became increasingly concerned by the language and attitudes expressed by

members of the organisation I had helped to start. The constant references to people who experience schizophrenia as 'sufferers' and 'victims' of illness seemed offensive to me. While I was the first to admit that schizophrenia had dominated my life for many years and that it could be a terrible disease, I also knew that I had only really made progress in my own recovery when I stopped seeing myself as a victim and relinquished the passive role in my treatment... Even for those of us facing great psychiatric disabilities, our souls can flower with hope.[6]

## Breaking the cycle of despair: the application of the new paradigm to employment

So can we break this self-fulfilling cycle of hopelessness, halt and reverse the journey to social exclusion and create the conditions where people can lead working lives when they are well? It has long been known that people with mental health problems are freer of symptoms and less prone to relapse if they have some constructive work activity to fill their days. Unfortunately this insight, when interpreted within the framework of the medical model, led to the concept of work as therapy rather than as paid employment. The revolutionary 1950s idea of creating industrial rehabilitation units put forward by pioneers such as Douglas Bennett at the Maudsley was rapidly subverted by general pessimism about patients' employment prospects. At first there was a clear intention to return people to the economy as well as to the community and some success in doing so. But rising levels of general unemployment and the lack of any clear relationship between what staff felt qualified to do and the requirements of a rapidly changing local labour market made the now renamed industrial therapy units alternatives to employment rather than stepping stones.

In the early 1990s some of us realised belatedly that for all our good intentions, almost no one in our schemes was getting a proper job – despite many being obviously capable and productive. Clearly we needed to change our practice but, more importantly, we had to change the way we thought about what we were doing – both service providers and users. We were, and to some extent still are, imprisoned by the dominant ways of thinking and the all-pervasive medical model. It is a hard thing to say but what follows from this is the serious charge that clinicians and other mental health workers have created a system that actually leads people further down the path of social exclusion and gets in the way of recovery and employment. Small wonder people call themselves 'survivors' of psychiatry when what they encounter is a system which, with the best of intentions, seeks to control them but offers little hope of recovery and a normal life.

## New ways of looking at evidence

The watchwords of current thinking on mental health services are that they must be 'evidence-based'. The problem with this is that evidence collected within the wrong theoretical paradigm will only serve to refine our understanding of that paradigm. The news that one particular drug has fewer debilitating effects than another is very useful if you are choosing between two forms of drug treatment. It does nothing to help people choose between different ways of managing mental distress or give any perspective on the role of long-term medication in people's lives.

Trying out new ways of thinking which challenge the dominant paradigm cannot be achieved only through research methods which take the usual way of thinking as a given, such as randomised controlled trials. For this to happen, we need a different kind of research which looks not simply at observable effects but also at the meaning of experience to different groups of people. Once we have a better understanding of the sometimes very different perceptions and experiences of service users, carers, employers and clinicians, we can start to look at the 'hard' evidence with new eyes. The question 'Does it work?' has to be answered in a context in which the further questions 'What does success mean; for whom; why; in what circumstances?' are also problematic.

In this book we present a body of evidence which explores questions of perception and experience as well as observable fact. By looking at the ways in which different actors in the mental health system see things and behave, we can set the (more circumscribed) evidence from trials of different forms of treatment or service into a new context. The questions we are trying to answer are very fundamental. Can the journey into disability and exclusion be halted? Is recovery possible? Can most people be employed if they want to? What are the conditions in which this is possible? Will they (and society) benefit if they are employed? These are all heavily value-based questions and depend for their answers on making values explicit. It is our view that only when we are able to talk honestly about basic values and reach some kind of consensus on what we are all trying to achieve will we be able to move forward. Once we are clear what we are trying to achieve, we can use different kinds of research methods to see whether particular interventions work and evaluate the evidence on what constitutes effective treatment and plan for the future.

So – the writers who have contributed to this volume have undertaken a challenging task. Studies have explored the understandings and employment aspirations of people who use mental health services. They have evaluated a service which aims to help people who are at risk of losing their jobs through mental ill health to remain in work. They have looked at the process of helping people back into employment after being out of the labour market for many years, seeking views on what works from employers, employees and support workers. They have looked at the struggle to introduce new ways of working into community mental health teams. And alongside these studies, writers who themselves use or have used mental health services provide powerful testimony of the importance of work in their lives and the struggle they have faced to stay in work. Others explore ways in which user-led services can help people facing multiple discrimination and cultural dissonance to hang on to their hopes and ambitions.

All these contributions are underpinned by a new paradigm. This puts the main focus of research enquiry and service delivery on intervening to halt and reverse the journey to exclusion. It assumes that the most important goal of mental health services is to provide as much treatment and support as necessary (and no more) for people to recover and lead ordinary lives as fully participating citizens. The questions for the reader are – if you look at the evidence for recovery and employment in the light of this new paradigm, does it make sense? Does it accord with or contradict the evidence from other kinds of research? Does it accord with or contradict your own experience?

If the new paradigm does make sense, we can begin to plan, deliver and evaluate future services within a shared conceptual universe in which we can at least feel that we are exploring the right questions. If it does not make sense then we must still go on exploring, because the present, predominantly medical, paradigm has failed to deliver either prevention or cure for long-term disability and exclusion, with tragic consequences for people with mental health problems, their friends, their carers and our whole society.

## An overview of the book

The current UK government is committed to improving employment opportunities for disabled people. Its mantra is 'Work for those who can, security for those who can't'. In many ways this is an admirable sentiment and a vast improvement on the neglect of disabled people's employment aspirations which preceded it. However, within the new paradigm this statement, dividing people into those who can and those who can't, is highly problematic. As Fiona Ford and colleagues succinctly put it:[7]

> While it is probably true that in the right circumstances almost everyone can work, it can equally be said that in the wrong circumstances almost nobody will.

With a nod in the direction of the government's mantra, Part 1 of this book is entitled 'Work with security when you can, security when you can't'. Together, the four chapters included here conclusively refute the prevailing myths about mental health and employment. The review in Chapter 1 of the research into who is and is not employable destroys the myth that it is the symptoms or severity of a person's mental distress that determine whether they are able to work. Rather, the most reliable indicator of employability is whether a person really wants a job. If they do, it is then for us to help them find one that suits their aspirations, skills and (self-defined) limitations.

But *do* people with mental health problems really want to work? As several contributors point out throughout the book, there is a widespread assumption among mental health professionals that for people who experience severe and enduring problems, work is simply off the agenda. Chapter 2 roundly scotches that myth by presenting the results of surveys that have gone beyond automatic assumptions to directly ask service users what they do want in the way of work, education and training. The resounding answer is that the majority of people do want some sort of work and they want help to find and keep a job that suits them. In Chapters 3 and 4, Mo Hutchison and Mary Nettle reinforce that message, describing how they have fought to keep working while experiencing severe mental distress, often with little support around work from mental health services.

One thing that becomes clear, though, is that people don't want employment at any price; hence our adjustment to the government's slogan in our title. A world of work in which people are expected to put up with intolerable stress, toxic working environments and chronic insecurity is what has driven many people we know over the edge. Our society is starting to be concerned about rising stress levels and work–life balance. If we are to hope to accommodate people who have looked despair in the face in our workforce, we need to adjust our thinking on what security *in* work means.

Part 2, 'Hitting the bottom and getting back up', takes up that theme in relation to how people who find themselves at the bottom of the slippery slope to long-term unemployment and social exclusion can be supported to make the journey back up to a fulfilling working life. To set the scene, in Chapters 5 and 6, Justine Schneider first reviews the international research into what works in enabling people who have long dropped out of the labour market to get back to work, and then examines how far along the road to putting the evidence into practice we are in the UK. The answer, unfortunately, is 'not very far'. Nevertheless, some excellent practice does exist, even if on a small scale. In Chapter 7 Jenny Secker and colleagues compare and contrast two very different approaches to employment support to reveal the centrality, if services are to be effective, of embracing a social understanding of recovery from mental ill health – an understanding based on the hope and expectation that with the right support, everyone who wants to work can find and keep a job.

What this research also reveals, however, is a gulf between employment support services and mental health services that severely hampers the good work being done. The research evidence outlined by Justine Schneider in Chapter 6 indicates that integrating vocational and mental health services produces the best outcomes and this is reinforced by a UK study of three organisational arrangements for the provision of employment support described in Chapter 8 by Patience Seebohm. While Patience's focus is on the benefits for both mental health professionals and service users of moving beyond the medical model to a truly community-oriented approach to mental healthcare, in Chapter 9 Rachel Perkins and Miles Rinaldi describe how the integration of vocational and mental health services has been achieved in South West London. From her perspective as a senior mental health service manager, Rachel provides eminently practical advice for others embarking on the process of integration, as well as highlighting the pitfalls she and her colleagues have encountered.

But what about those people whose confidence has fallen so low that at the moment they can't contemplate working, though they wish they could? And what about people deterred by fear of stigmatisation and harsh treatment from using any mental health services? In Chapters 10 and 11 Graham Cockshutt and Paul Grey describe the achievements of two user-led vocational services established as part of a Department of Health funded initiative, Unlocking Potential, that aimed to find innovative ways to support people in these situations. While Graham's focus is the establishment of a self-help group (though he has reservations about this term!) of service users in Sheffield, Paul describes how he was able to support young black men, a group often fearful of mental health services, to work towards achieving their aspirations in London. As people with experience of using mental health services themselves, it is clear that Graham and Paul also gained much from their work on these projects.

Part 2 ends with a further contribution from three people with experience of using both mental health and vocational services. Having previously received employment support themselves, John Marshall and Jo Shenton now work at Rethink Graphics, an employment project in Brentwood, Essex, supporting other people to achieve their aspirations. From his perspective as employment coordinator, John describes what he has found effective in enabling people to gain confidence, identify their goals and achieve them, bringing to life the rather drier accounts in the research literature with which Part 2 began. Jo then tells us the 'story so far' of her journey to recovery, revealing not only how important work and creativity are on that journey but also how a sense of humour helps. Finally, their co-contributor, Richard Watts, describes his own 'employment adventures' and how the support he receives from Rethink Graphics is indeed enabling him to rethink his goals and make use of his writing skills in a very different career from that on which he originally embarked.

So far so good, but why must people who need to use mental health services endure the pain and despair of sliding to the bottom of the slippery slope, experiencing the erosion of hope often for years? As the wealth of literature reviewed in Parts 1 and 2 illustrates, supporting these people back up the slope has been the main focus of attention among writers and researchers in this field. Yet when people first come into contact with mental health services it is more likely than not that they will be in employment or education. Can we not help them to keep their job or college place or support them back into work quickly if they are already on the slippery slope? Recently, the focus of research and service development has begun to move 'upstream' to address these questions and this is our own focus in Part 3, 'Avoiding the slippery slope'.

In Chapter 13, Tina Thomas and Jenny Secker review the international research into how people experiencing mental health problems can be helped to keep their job or find one that suits them better without first dropping out of the labour market. The same authors then present the results of their evaluation of an innovative job retention service in the West of England, which illustrates the potential of intervening early to prevent job loss.

That potential is reinforced in Chapter 15 by Miles Rinaldi and Rachel Perkins, who again draw on their experience in South West London to argue the case for early intervention and to describe the results they have achieved by providing ready access to vocational support both within community mental health teams and within a service for young people experiencing a first episode of psychosis.

Finally we try to draw some theoretical and practical conclusions from our explorations of the new paradigm. Our journeys take us to some places that people schooled in the 'illness' model of mental distress and disorder may find surprising. Among other things, they have led us inexorably to a redefinition of the relationship between service users and mental health professionals – a redefinition that calls into question basic assumptions about roles, power and control of resources. But this is to anticipate – for now let us express the hope that you enjoy reading this book as much as we have enjoyed writing it.

# References

1 Kruger A (2000) Schizophrenia, recovery and hope. *Psychiatric Rehabilitation Journal.* **24**(1): 29–37.

2 Kraepelin E (1912) *Clinical Psychiatry: a textbook for students and physicians* (trans. A Diefendorf). Macmillan, New York.

3 Harding C, Brooks G, Ashikaga T *et al.* (1987) The Vermont longitudinal study of persons with severe mental illness, I : Methodology, study sample and overall status 32 years later. *American Journal of Psychiatry.* **144**(6): 718–26.

4 Harrison G, Hopper K, Craig T *et al.* (2001) Recovery from psychotic illness: a 15- and 25-year international follow up study. *British Journal of Psychiatry.* **178**: 506–17.

5 Harding C, cited in Pierce C (1994) Longest ever schizophrenia studies indicate high recovery rate. *Clinical Psychiatry News.* **August**: 8.

6 Champ S, cited in Barker P, Campbell P and Davidson B (1999) *From the Ashes of Experience: reflections on madness, survival and growth.* Whurr, London.

7 Ford F, Ford J and Dowrick C (2000) Welfare to work: the role of general practice. Discussion paper. *British Journal of General Practice.* **50**: 497–500.

# Part 1

# Work with security when you can, security when you can't

# Chapter 1

# Sheep and goats: new thinking on employability

Bob Grove and Helen Membrey

## Introduction

There are a number of deeply embedded assumptions within mental health services about the willingness and ability of people with severe and enduring mental health problems to enter the labour market.

One is that people with mental health problems do not want to work. In fact, significant numbers make obtaining work one of the main goals of their recovery journey. In the spring of 2003, the UK Labour Force Survey showed that 35% of people with mental health problems who were economically inactive wanted to work. In fact, this is probably an underestimate. As Patience Seebohm and Jenny Secker demonstrate in the next chapter, surveys that have asked people about both their current and longer term aspirations show that the majority of people identified as having severe and enduring mental health problems want to return to employment eventually. Many service users have at some point in their lives been told that they will never work again, presumably with the intention of reconciling them to their condition and relieving them of the worry of earning a living. Whatever the intention, it is a profoundly discouraging message and can feel like a life sentence of poverty and second-class citizenship.

Another assumption and the focus of this chapter is also connected to the wish of clinicians to be what they would consider realistic. Their argument in my experience goes something like this: 'Of course, we know that not everyone will be able to work so we cannot put too much emphasis on employment and we have to find something for the others to do'. One counter-argument for this is that as we have never really tried to get a job for everyone who wants to work, we do not know how many are likely to be unemployable. We cannot know what we don't know.

However, there is within the assumption a testable proposition. If we accept that for the time being services are not available to support everyone who might want a job, and then predict who is likely to be employable, we can put them in employment programmes and find the others something else to do. In fact, a considerable amount of research has gone into finding ways of sorting out the employable sheep from the unemployable goats.

But is it possible to assess who is likely to be able to hold down a job? Are there personal characteristics or indicators in a person's medical or social or employment history that make it possible to select those who should go into vocational programmes? When we reviewed the research evidence, it became apparent that there are very few.

## Research findings on employability

Research in the vocational rehabilitation field over the last few decades has been predominantly North American, driven largely by a concern to find out which service users will respond best to vocational interventions on the basis of their individual characteristics. Clinical factors, social skills, employment history and a range of psychological factors have all been examined. Let's look at the evidence for each in turn.

## Clinical factors

The clinical factors that researchers have examined in relation to their implications for employability include diagnosis, symptoms and hospitalisation history. Where diagnosis is concerned, there is strong evidence that a person's psychiatric diagnosis does not affect their ability to succeed in vocational programmes.[1] Very few studies have found a link between either diagnosis or severity of impairment and employment retention, a conclusion confirmed by an extensive review.[2]

On the issue of how symptoms might affect service users' ability to work, there is conflicting and equivocal evidence. Some studies suggest that symptoms do not prevent service users participating in employment programmes and improving their vocational performance.[2–5] William Anthony found evidence from another nine studies from the 1960s, 1970s and early 1980s all confirming that 'there appear to be no symptoms or symptom patterns that are consistently related to individual work performance'.[2] Nevertheless, it has been argued that the more severe a service user's symptoms, the more impaired their work performance and for that reason people are often cautious about allowing service users to work until their symptoms improve. Symptoms have been seen as predictors of social skills and work skills. Others, however, argue that assessments of symptoms have been too generic to pick up the relationship between these different areas of functioning.[6,7] They have suggested that work performance and symptoms are distinct but interrelated areas and that there is a need to understand how specific symptoms affect particular areas of functioning. Although more research is clearly needed to clarify this rather confusing picture, an important point about these studies of symptom effects is that ratings must be made concurrently with work activity as these are more powerful predictors than those recorded at intake to a programme. In other words, symptoms vary considerably over time and should not be used to select people into vocational programmes because it is not possible to predict their impact in a real work context.

In addition to or instead of symptoms, researchers have looked at service users' clinical background in terms of how many lifetime hospitalisations they have had or the length and date of their most recent hospitalisation.[4, 8] One study revealed that being recently hospitalised does have an independent effect on work status, separate from the known effect of reducing service users' functioning levels.[4] However, as the authors point out, it is impossible to pin down the nature of this relationship. Does the effect of entering a hospital in recent history diminish employment outcomes because of the stigma and disruption it causes or is it that work lessens the likelihood of being hospitalised in the first place?

Furthermore, there is considerable evidence that participation in work activity can have long-term beneficial effects on clinical outcomes such as symptoms, medication, compliance and relapse rates.[9-12] It could be that returning to valued, adult roles has a positive impact on service users' self-esteem and their ability to manage their own illness, thus reducing symptoms.

What is clear is that the evidence does not strongly favour the use of symptom assessments, diagnosis or hospitalisation history to exclude service users from vocational programmes.

## Social skills

Most studies show that social skills have only a small or non-significant relationship with vocational outcomes.[2] While some have argued that the ability to get along with others in the workplace plays an important part in vocational success, the best way to assess these skills remains largely unresolved. There is evidence to suggest that when skills are tested generically in artificial environments, the results do not translate easily to the real world and this could be one explanation why traditional measures of social skills have not produced significant results.[13,14]

However, in one study the authors found that social skills improved significantly after as little as 17 weeks when service users were placed in real work situations.[6] They explained this in terms of the increase in self-esteem and confidence that comes from having a productive work role, from overcoming fears of rejection, adjusting to expected social behaviours in the workplace and working alongside regular colleagues. As with symptoms, if social skills can be enhanced through work participation, then service users who initially perform poorly in this domain should not be excluded from vocational interventions.

## Employment history

On the face of it, the most promising predictor of future vocational performance appears to be the amount of previous work experience people have.[1,2,15-17] Although researchers have used different definitions to measure work experience (e.g. length of whole career, number of jobs over a career, length of different jobs, date of last employment), overall there is strong evidence that people with more work experience benefit more from vocational programmes than people with little or no work experience. In one review, for example, employment history accounted for as much as 53% of the variance in vocational outcomes.[18]

However, several more recent studies have incorporated newly recognised variables in more complex research designs. These studies indicate that psychological factors are more important than employment history. For instance, one study found that although both employment history and symptomatology were initially associated with vocational outcomes, these connections disappeared when service users' 'self-efficacy', or belief about how effective they could be in taking control of their lives, was taken into account.[19] A belief in personal effectiveness was what made the difference, not previous employment or symptoms. Similarly, there is some evidence that being goal-oriented is more important than how much work experience one has. Employment history did not predict outcomes in one study and the authors explained this in terms of how they had selected their research sample.[20]

Once again, the conclusion to be drawn from the evidence is that service users should not be excluded from vocational programmes on the grounds of limited work experience. It is belief in oneself and motivation that count. Some further psychological factors that have been examined in their own right are considered next.

## Psychological factors

Alongside self-efficacy and being goal-oriented, work attitudes, work expectations and motivation to work have been shown to be important for vocational outcomes.

Several studies have found correlations between work adjustment skills and vocational performance.[2,15,21,22] It has not always been clear which aspects of 'work adjustment' are critical but some studies indicate that the most important is a 'strong feeling about the importance of work as a source of pride and accomplishment'.[1,4,23] However, here we have the familiar problem with direction of causality: do positive feelings about work accomplishments reflect a stronger motivation to gain and sustain work or could it be that having a job heightens these feelings? In other studies, positive expectations about obtaining work made a significant contribution to participation in vocational projects.[24,25]

One of the most interesting conclusions to come out of the research to date stems from the in-depth study of barriers to work for employed and unemployed service users carried out by Alex Braitman and colleagues.[24] Although the study identified a wide range of barriers, including entitlements, anxiety about work and substance abuse problems, the results also indicate that motivation may override all other barriers to work. In light of this, the authors argue that barriers identified by earlier research may only be significant because of the way in which they affect service users' motivational levels. It will probably come as no surprise, for example, that pay is an important motivating factor. In one study the effect of returning to unpaid work placements after experiencing competitive paid work demotivated project participants and their work skills declined.[11] Frequent job loss and unsuccessful outcomes at work can, also unsurprisingly, lower service users' motivation to pursue their employment goals. As with other individual characteristics, however, the causes of poor motivation are ambiguous. Is it that repeated failures in the workplace lead to poor motivation or that lower motivational levels reduce work skills?

Coming back to self-efficacy, a few researchers have looked specifically at this as a predictor of future vocational performance rather than comparing it with employment history.[19] These studies show that people with higher levels of self-efficacy tend to persevere longer and that as they experience mastery over a situation, their sense of effectiveness increases further. In contrast, those with low self-efficacy tend to avoid situations and environments that they feel they can't cope with, further reinforcing their view of themselves as not possessing the necessary skills to succeed.

In another study, self-efficacy was found to be important in the long-term success of rehabilitation.[10] Changes in vocational status seemed to affect self-esteem and life satisfaction by modifying feelings of self-efficacy. Enhancing self-efficacy may therefore lead to positive vocational effects.

## So can we predict who will be employable?

What emerges strongly from the research evidence we have reviewed is that there is no case for discouraging service users from pursuing their vocational goals on the basis of their diagnosis, symptoms, hospitalisation history, level of social functioning or employment history. In fact, working may actually reduce symptoms, improve social skills and reduce the likelihood of being hospitalised. Obviously, it also contributes accumulating work experience for the CV. An important point to come out of Braitman and colleagues' study of barriers to work[24] was that service users who were in jobs were experiencing difficulties but were overcoming them. They were able to work despite the side effects of medication, symptoms, anxiety and so forth.

The evidence for psychological factors, such as motivation and a person's sense of how effective they are, is more consistent and powerful. Interestingly, these factors are consistent with the 'recovery model' that has recently come to prominence in the North American literature.[26] In this context, recovery is seen as a process of recovering social roles and ambitions that have been lost through the experience of mental illness and becoming a patient. Ideas about recovery therefore focus on how service users can be empowered to manage their own illness and live the kind of lives they choose. But does this mean that we should exclude from vocational programmes service users whose levels of motivation and self-belief are low? We think not. As William Anthony argues, these psychological characteristics can themselves be fostered through engagement with appropriate vocational services and should not, therefore, be used to judge who is ready for employment.[2]

> The more reasonable and less exclusionary acceptance factors may be an interested and ready individual and a relevant vocational rehabilitation intervention.

## Conclusion

The argument that we can predict who will be employable and therefore decide who should be included in vocational programmes is not supported by the research evidence. It follows that every person who uses mental health services should be offered the chance of employment if that is what they want. The only indicator we need to worry about is whether they want to work and even this is not fixed for all time. The research shows that experiencing some success at work is likely to enhance motivation, skills and self-confidence. People change and what is true at one point in a person's life may not be true at others.

We must therefore keep an open mind about an individual's employability and be alert for the moment when it feels right to them to move forward and take the risk of going for a job. Or as Bob Drake once said, when asked by a student how he thought people should be selected for employment programmes, 'We select anyone who holds their hand up'.[27]

We must also shift the focus from the individual to the type of help they are offered. In several of the studies which set out to test service users' characteristics in relation to vocational success, researchers discovered that the different approaches of the service agencies involved seemed to play a far more significant part in employment outcomes.[3,23,28] What really matters, then, is not how the individual appears to us when they first embark on the journey to employment but how well we help them overcome the barriers they face. The question of what kind of services do help people find and keep a job is the focus of Part 2 of this book.

# References

1 Bybee D, Mowbray C and McCrohan N (1996) Towards zero exclusion in vocational opportunities for persons with psychiatric disabilities: prediction of service receipt in a hybrid vocational/case management service programme. *Psychiatric Rehabilitation Journal.* **19**(4): 15–27.

2 Anthony W (1994) Characteristics of people with psychiatric disabilities that are predictive of entry into the rehabilitation process and successful employment outcomes. *Psychosocial Rehabilitation Journal.* **17**(3): 3–14.

3 Drake R, Becker D, Biesanz J *et al.* (1996) Day treatment versus supported employment for persons with severe mental illness: a replication study. *Psychiatric Services.* **47**(10): 1125–7.

4 Mowbray C, Bybee D, Harris S *et al.* (1995) Predictors of work status and future work orientation in people with a psychiatric disability. *Psychiatric Rehabilitation Journal.* **19**(2): 17–28.

5 Smith T, Rio J, Hull J *et al.* (1998) The Rehabilitation Readiness Determination Profile: a needs assessment for adults with severe mental illness. *Psychiatric Rehabilitation Journal.* **21**(4): 380–7.

6 Lysaker P and Bell M (1995) Work performance over time for people with schizophrenia. *Psychiatric Rehabilitation Journal.* **18**(3): 141–5.

7 Smith T, Rio J, Hull J *et al.* (1997) Differential effects of symptoms on rehabilitation and adjustment in people with schizophrenia. *Psychiatric Rehabilitation Journal.* **21**(2): 141–3.

8 Rogers E, MacDonald-Wilson K, Danley K *et al.* (1997) A process analysis of supported employment services for persons with serious psychiatric disability: implications for programme design. *Journal of Vocational Rehabilitation.* **8**(3): 232–42.

9 Anthony W, Rogers E, Cohen M *et al.* (1995) Relationships between psychiatric symptomatology, work skills and future vocational performance. *Psychiatric Services.* **46**(4): 353–8.

10 Arns P and Linney J (1993) Work, self and life satisfaction for persons with severe and persistent mental disorders. *Psychosocial Rehabilitation Journal.* **17**(2): 63–80.

11 Bell M, Milstein R and Lysaker P (1993) Pay and participation in work activity: clinical benefits for clients with schizophrenia. *Psychosocial Rehabilitation Journal.* **17**(2): 173–7.

12 Lehman A (1995) Vocational rehabilitation in schizophrenia. *Schizophrenia Bulletin.* **21**: 645–6.

13 Cook J and Pickett S (1994) Recent trends in vocational rehabilitation for people with psychiatric disability. *American Rehabilitation.* **20**(4): 2–12.

14 Rogan P and Hagner D (1990) Vocational evaluation in supported employment.

*Journal of Rehabilitation.* **Jan–March**: 45–51.

15 Anthony W and Jansen M (1984) Predicting the vocational capacity of the chronically mentally ill. *American Psychologist.* **39**: 537–44.

16 Bond G (1992) Vocational rehabilitation. In: R Liberman (ed.) *Handbook of Psychiatric Rehabilitation.* Macmillan, New York.

17 Xie H, Dain B, Becker D *et al.* (1997) Job tenure among persons with severe mental illness. *Rehabilitation Counselling Bulletin.* **40**(4): 230–9.

18 Anthony W, Cohen M and Farkas M (1990) *Psychiatric Rehabilitation.* Boston University Center for Psychiatric Rehabilitation, Boston.

19 Regenold M, Sherman M and Fenzel M (1999) Getting back to work: self-efficacy as a predictor of employment outcome. *Psychiatric Rehabilitation Journal.* **22**(4): 361–7.

20 Rogers E, Anthony W, Toole J *et al.* (1991) Vocational outcomes following psychosocial rehabilitation: a longitudinal study of three programs. *Journal of Vocational Rehabilitation.* **1**(3): 21–9.

21 Bond G and Friedmeyer M (1987) Predictive validity of situational assessment at a psychiatric rehabilitation center. *Rehabilitation Psychology.* **32**(2): 99–112.

22 Bryson G, Bell M, Lysaker P *et al.* (1997) The Work Behaviour Inventory: a scale for the assessment of work behavior of people with severe mental illness. *Psychiatric Rehabilitation Journal.* **20**(4): 47–55.

23 Blankertz L and Robinson S (1996) Adding a vocational focus to mental health rehabilitation. *Psychiatric Services.* **47**(11): 1216–22.

24 Braitman A, Counts P, Davenport R *et al.* (1995) Comparison of barriers to employment for unemployed and employed clients in a case management programme: an exploratory study. *Psychiatric Rehabilitation Journal.* **19**(1): 3–8.

25 Rutman I (1994) How psychiatric disability expresses itself as a barrier to employment. *Psychosocial Rehabilitation Journal.* **17**(3): 15–36.

26 Anthony W (1993) Recovery from mental illness: the guiding vision of the mental health system in the 1990s. *Psychosocial Rehabilitation Journal.* **16**(4): 11–23.

27 Drake R (2003) *Recent research on vocational rehabilitation for adults with severe mental illness.* Proceedings of the 6th European Union of Supported Employment Conference, 21–23 May, 2003, Helsinki, Finland.

28 Bond G, Drake R, Mueser K *et al.* (1997) An update on supported employment for people with severe mental illness. *Psychiatric Services.* **48**(3): 335–46.

# Chapter 10

# Unlocking Potential in Sheffield

Graham Cockshutt

## Introduction

Unlocking Potential was a three-year initiative funded by the Department of Health. The aim of the initiative was to develop employment services led by mental health service users in two communities. In the next chapter Paul Grey describes the project that was established in East London to help young black men achieve their aspirations. I was asked to contribute this chapter because I coordinate the other project that was established in Sheffield.

A central idea behind the Unlocking Potential initiative was that the two projects should develop in line with the needs of local service users and for this reason they worked in rather different ways. In Sheffield, we established a 'self-help' group to support people with mental health problems towards employment. As Paul explains in his chapter, this approach was less appropriate for the young black men with whom he worked, so one-to-one work became more important in East London.

One of the difficulties with the term 'self-help' is that for me it generates uncomfortable associations, not in a Freudian sense (just in case my psychiatrist reads this) but in the sense of self-harm, self-medication, self-service. They are all activities that you do to or for yourself. Looking at what has been written about self-help, it's clear that the definitions available are as numerous as self-help groups themselves. One of the most frequently quoted is this definition offered by Katz and Bender:[1]

> ...voluntary, small group structures for mutual aid in the accomplishment of a specific purpose. They are usually formed by peers who have come together for mutual assistance in satisfying a common need, overcoming a common handicap or life-disrupting problem and bringing about desired social and/or personal change (p.9).

Further definitions include 'created social units [involving] new social forms of coping, lay autonomy and the humanisation of health care'[2] and lists of specifications such as this one from Gartner and Riessman.[3]

1. Self-help groups always involve face-to-face interactions.
2. The origin of the self-help group is usually spontaneous.
3. Personal participation is extremely important since bureaucratisation is the enemy of the self-help group.
4. The members agree on and engage in activities.

5. The group fulfils the need for a reference group, a point of connection and identification with others and a base for activity.
6. Typically the groups start from a condition of powerlessness (p. 613).

Other authors have amended, amplified or reinterpreted these commonly cited definitions but the purpose of including them here is really to show you that there is no one definition of self-help and consequently each group has to establish its own. For my own part, I have never been good at self-help and I am not convinced that the term itself is appropriate. When you are unwell, with any sort of illness, the ability to make rational and informed decisions about almost anything disappears very quickly. The only time I offer advice to people is to tell them not to make any major decisions when they are unwell. The problem, of course, is that all too frequently the option is removed from you anyway and any sense of control is vested in others. So for me, although the term 'self-help' is rather problematic, the idea that it starts from a condition of being powerless is very much in keeping with how service users can feel. As I hope to show as I describe the work of Unlocking Potential in Sheffield, other ideas put forward in the definitions are also useful, particularly mutual help and autonomy.

From the start of Unlocking Potential in Sheffield in the summer of 2001, I realised that my own experience of an enduring mental health problem would inevitably influence the running of the project and that it was going to become a peer support group and not just a self-help group. For me this gets to the essence of what can be achieved by, and the real dichotomy of, self-help groups. Let me explain. Self-help means helping yourself or, in the wider sense, a group of people helping themselves. In many cases, though, the power base is still vested in others because terms of reference and finance are controlled externally: jump through the hoops or you get nothing. Many self-help groups emerge from previously established groups and are deemed 'self-help' only because their members are service users. For people to really benefit, there has to be autonomy.

## Our aims

So what does the Unlocking Potential group do? How is it constructed? How does it help people get back into employment? Most importantly, does it work? Before I answer those questions, I should define employment. For me, employment is any meaningful activity that a person undertakes. You may think at this point that I've been working with occupational therapists for too long but for me, employment is not about payment, it is about worth. The individual needs to feel that whatever they are doing is worthwhile and not just a 'time filler'.

One of the basic precepts of Unlocking Potential in Sheffield is therefore that people should not be written off by others or themselves. We aim to encourage people who have experienced mental health problems to resume a profitable, fulfilling life, achieving *what they* want as individuals and achieving it *when they* want to. That said, Unlocking Potential acknowledges that people who have, or have had, mental health problems often experience difficulties in finding, getting and maintaining the right employment openings that all too frequently people exclude them from. The chance of securing and maintaining employment can be improved with the right support but much of that support needs to come from people who have experienced similar difficulties and not from well-meaning others.

All too often we attempt to hide our mental illness from everyone because of the probability of a negative reaction from friends, employers, prospective employers or the general public. The consequence of this is that we are often made to feel guilty about our illness, almost as if it is a moral judgement. Unlocking Potential aims to address this stigma and discrimination, particularly where it exists in the workplace, by promoting its replacement with a more realistic view. Employers (and the general public) need to be encouraged to see the real potential of people with personal experience of mental health difficulties.

We believe that the expert role of people who have experienced or are experiencing mental health problems can be used to help others avoid making the same mistakes when seeking employment. This could significantly reduce the stress of returning to some form of work or of achieving the ambitions that we are all entitled to have. An overriding objective of the group is to utilise the expertise gained by service users who have returned to work or taken up voluntary activities in order to benefit others. Those involved are provided with training and personal development to further support them with the practicalities of assisting other service users.

## Establishing the group

In Sheffield, Unlocking Potential set about establishing a peer support group to promote employment, voluntary activities and training. An important issue for me is to make sure that the group is kept small, with no more than six or eight people involved. At times, up to 15 people have been involved but a core group of eight service users with the skills, attitude and aptitude to develop user-led activities has emerged. Keeping the group small is not about elitism but about understanding the needs of individuals. All too often in large groups factions can develop and this, in turn, leads to conflict. There are times when an element of conflict can be healthy but it can also be disruptive and destructive. As a fully paid-up member of the 'self-preservation society', I felt that it was a variable I would try to eliminate. A smaller group also makes it more feasible to provide in-depth training and develop personal plans and objectives. This is important because the Unlocking Potential group consists of a variety of people, some of whom have worked and some of whom have never worked. Some have jobs that they are returning to, others have no idea what they are going to do. The common factor for all of us is a sense of wanting to help each other, and ourselves, to move forward. The small group means that a sense of bonding takes place quite quickly and this has become an important factor in how the group has developed.

At an early stage we decided what training we needed and how it would benefit us. The training we identified fell into two broad categories: we needed information about certain issues and we needed to improve some of our skills. On the basis of the information needs we identified, we were provided with training on the welfare benefits system, the voluntary sector and employment training groups. In terms of improving our skills, we had training in giving presentations and running groups, and all members also followed a course that started them on the road to becoming qualified trainers. This was important because it helped to boost confidence and although some people felt unwell, because of the support they were getting from each other, they continued through with the course and completed it.

## Supporting each other

The support network that has been constructed among members is very important. It isn't a link between the individual members of the group, although there may be specific bonds that tie them together. Rather, it is the intergroup dynamics that allow a person to feel that they can contact any member of the group if they feel they need support. This means that, at all times, support is only a telephone call away.

What is also vital is the way in which the group has been constructed with a good mix of people who are at various stages of recovery. It would have seemed inconceivable to me three years ago to ask a person who has not worked for a long time for advice on my work situation but in the group I do exactly that. The result is quite frequently a more realistic view of the situation and comments that may not be directly opposed to what I am thinking but that certainly makes me reconsider what I am planning to do. Without this injection of realism, it is quite possible that an individual could go off along their own path and feel unsupported again. Returning to work necessitates support and a strong support network if it is to be successful. The Unlocking Potential group provides such a network and although it is not complete in itself, it does establish a good basis and, more importantly, a learning environment for the individual.

The support people receive from the group has been generated mainly through something I haven't mentioned yet, the social aspect of what we do. We meet together for a meal or a social drink twice a month or so and talk through various issues, looking at what might be coming up, planning out future work, thinking about how to support each other, what help anyone needs. All of these are seen as important aspects that are discussed in a relaxed, social atmosphere, not in the formality of a meeting room in an NHS hospital. To some people this might not seem important but for me, and for the group, it is the single most important factor. It shows people that they are entitled to have a social life and that social life can also play an important role in shaping their future. It has led to us looking at what research we could undertake, how we could generate income, what training we are all doing and how that could be tied in together, and how we could develop the group to spread the ideals and beliefs that we hold much more widely. Contact between individuals, depending on their needs at any one time, might be more frequent, sometimes daily or weekly.

# The role of mental health professionals

One of the questions constantly asked by the members of the group, and one that I admit I ask myself, is 'What is the role of the health professional in this process?'. The group is, by its nature, a group of people with similar needs helping each other and learning to help themselves. Where then does the professional fit into this? Returning to the autonomy issue I raised earlier, professionals have never been involved in the organisation or support networks of the Unlocking Potential group. This has not been the case in other self-help groups that I have been involved with. For example, the original Sheffield Hearing Voices group was set up by a professional who was inevitably involved in the group. One of the problems with this is that the methods, language and jargon used by professionals can result in an inability to really communicate with the service users they set out to assist. Equally, the group may adopt a similar language and consequently move away from their original intention of helping each other, becoming more of an intellectualised discussion group rather than a peer support group.

That is not to say that there is no role for professionals in the initiation of groups but there is a high risk of their role becoming patronising and of the group becoming nothing more than one of the numerous groups that service users are expected to attend in order to facilitate their recovery. There does come a point within self-help groups where confidence may deteriorate and the involvement of a professional is seen as legitimising that particular group. It is certainly true that in the Unlocking Potential group we have, on occasions, sought help from professionals in order to confirm that what we are doing or attempting is correct. It is important to emphasise, however, that this is not because the professionals involved have been trying to 'take over' or that they have been trying to dictate what happens. It is more a case of members seeking reassurance. As coordinator of the group, I have to accept that there are times when my knowledge is lacking. The professional can be asked to provide information, training, advice on organisation and, possibly, on public relation skills. In addition, many of the skills professionals have in establishing groups revolve around aims and evaluation and whilst self-help groups may not relish formalised aims and evaluation, I have come to realise that these are an important part of the development of both the group and the individuals within it. Clear aims and a clear way of measuring the achievement of those aims can be important, especially when the members of the group change or the dynamics of the group change as a result of an increase in size or external pressures.

The role of the professional can almost be seen as that of a supporting actor. They have no responsibility within the group or for the group. In an ideal world that, of course, would be how it would work in all mental health services. The reality is somewhat different but as part of its work, the Unlocking Potential group is attempting to break down the barriers between health professionals and service users. Cooperation with professionals has been an important part of the development of both the group and the individuals within it. They have come to see professionals not as opponents or enemies or barriers but as people who can help, guide and be involved in both their own development and the development of the group. Professionals are not considered as 'consultants' to the group – a term which generates a feeling of disempowerment for the individual, especially given the medical context in which we usually meet consultants – but as colleagues and as equal participants. More importantly, their involvement is controlled by the group, through invitations to join our social evenings and this is, in itself, an empowering position which generates confidence in people. Interestingly, when health professionals realise that we are having a social evening, they are often very keen to be invited. This may well be because it gives them an opportunity to escape an oppressive environment that they feel constrains what they can say and how they can express themselves. It would also be true to say that the sense of control that this gives the group is quite pleasing because they know that it is their choice and they are in control. It is marvellous what happens when the tables turn and how much pleasure these little things can give people!

I should add that the involvement of professionals has helped to encourage a much more balanced approach and this has been important. All too often service users, and myself especially, have been known to take a stand which, though morally and logically justifiable, is pragmatically unfeasible. This, of course, does not diminish in any way the validity of the stance, but sticking to it does tend to put you into conflict with the authorities. Working with professionals makes you aware of the parameters that people have to work within and the constraints many workers feel are placed on them.

At this stage you may well be thinking, what on earth has this got to do with a self-help group that aims to support people towards employment? In fact, it has a lot to do with the development of the individual and the way in which we perceive ourselves. By becoming aware of the parameters and the restrictions that people are sometimes placed under, be they financial, managerial or governmental, service users begin to accept the realities of the working world and to come to terms with the fact that ambition has to be counterbalanced with pragmatism.

## My own role

From how I've described the group so far, it may sound as if I am detached from it, running it but not part of it. This is far from the case. I have benefited from it more than I could ever have expected. Working part-time and running the group as well meant that I was under some pressure. Training commitments meant that the pressure increased and my free time was decreasing quite rapidly. Who better to tell you openly that things are beginning to go wrong than another service user? Or in this case two or three, each giving me the same message: practise what you preach, slow down, cut down your commitments. Most importantly, these things haven't been said to me in a way that makes me feel I'm being ordered about. They've been said in a spirit of advice, support and concern. Mind you, empathetic as they are, my fellow service users are not noted for their subtlety!

As I said earlier, the group provides me with an invaluable support network, in terms of not only providing advice on employment issues but also being able to understand the realities of an illness. What group members do not do is dwell on problems; what they try to do is to suggest solutions or coping strategies they have used and think might work for others.

Being involved in the group is also a humbling exercise. It puts your own difficulties into perspective and makes you appreciate more the positive aspects that exist. Self-help groups help you to develop self-confidence. Initially, this may only be within your own particular group but those learning points can be used in a wider environment. Self-help groups can help you become an educator. This is not compulsory, of course, but many people do find that because of their involvement they actually want to go out and talk with other people. In short, the group provides friendship, a contact point and a learning base from which the individual can develop. I have probably learned more from self-help groups than I have from any other source. I am kept in place and my feet frequently return to earth with a resounding jolt.

## So what have we achieved?

But I hear the sound of questions. Has it got people back to work? What are the short-term outcomes? Is it cost-effective? Well, on the work front all eight people who formed the core of the group are now doing something, whether it is paid or not (the majority are in paid jobs). With only one exception, all the members of the group have established self-help groups of their own in different spheres. Interestingly, they still come back to base and participate in the group in which they were founder members. Pragmatism is at the fore and this helps everyone in the group, not just me, to develop. The confidence people gain is, almost certainly, something that they will carry with them for the rest of their lives.

On the research front, we have become involved in research on voice hearing, on voluntary activities and, more recently, on the role of occupational therapists. Further training to support us in this covers the areas of voice hearing, paranoia, stigma and discrimination, the voluntary sector and the importance of employment to the recovery of an individual.

As regards cost-effectiveness, I couldn't possibly comment. I find it impossible to put a price on recovery although I am equally sure that somewhere there is a formula to work it out. What I do know is that the group has a waiting list and health professionals see it as a valuable and successful way of working. That is not to say that we can be complacent. The group has taught me that recovery and support go hand in hand with respect and honesty. It has also shown me that real empowerment only takes place when we take control for ourselves.

## References

1 Katz A and Bender E (eds) (1976) *The Strength in Us: self-help groups and the modern world.* Franklin Watts, London.
2 Kickbush I and Hatch S (eds) (1983) *Self-help and Health in Europe: new approaches to care.* World Health Organisation, Copenhagen.
3 Gartner A and Riessman F (1982) Self-help and mental health. *Hospital and Community Psychiatry.* **33**: 631–5.

# Chapter 11

# Unlocking the potential of young black men

Paul Grey

## Introduction

In the previous chapter, Graham Cockshutt described the Unlocking Potential project that was established in Sheffield. As he explained, both projects were part of a three-year initiative funded by the Department of Health, although the project in London took longer to shape than the one in Sheffield because we needed to spend longer exploring what would work best there. As project development worker for Unlocking Potential in London, my task in this chapter is to describe our work in providing peer support to young African and Caribbean men who have mental health issues and want to move on in the areas of training and 'real' work. First, though, let me tell you a little of my own story so you can see why I wanted to take on this challenge.

> Dear Sir or Madam, I am writing to you concerning my receipt of incapacity benefit. As of the 25th October 1999, I declare myself fit for work. I will also become self-employed from the same date. Thank you very much for your assistance over the years. Please can any excess funds or relevant information be sent to me at your convenience. Yours faithfully, Paul Grey

This is the text of a letter I sent to the benefits department in 1999, after spending over 10 years in and out of the mental health system. My problems had come to a head when I was 20 years old and just coming to the end of a four-year plumbing apprenticeship with the council. My parents were away for three months and without them around I had stopped eating properly. I also had a lot of major decisions to deal with, one of which was to decide whether to stay with the council. They wanted me to stay but I decided to go. I will never forget the week that I was sitting in the manager's office. He was pleading with me to give them a chance and then the following week I was sitting in the benefits office, seeking benefits. With all this newfound time on my hands and no way of getting my previously good eating habits back into order, my health started to deteriorate. To cut a long story short I soon ended up in a psychiatric ward. I realised then that I had made a big mistake, I did not want to be there; I wanted to be plumbing with the council.

In my own life, it was encouraging words of hope that worked for me and my role with Unlocking Potential was to offer inspiration, hope, coping strategies and general support to other young black men. Before I say more about the work of the project, I'll look at the problems for young black men and what I see as their causes and effects.

## Problems, causes and effects

My mother has always said that when your hand is in a lion's mouth, be careful how you take it out. The lion is the mental health system and when it gets its teeth into you, it won't let you go. As a recent study at the Sainsbury Centre for Mental Health highlights, the experience of black people in the mental health system is distinctly different from that of white people.[1] Here are some facts and figures that explain just how different the experience is.

- Black men, and especially young men, are more likely to be given a diagnosis of schizophrenia and less likely to have a diagnosis of depression.[2]
- Black men are more likely than other groups to come into contact with services via the police and the criminal justice system.[3]
- They are overrepresented in locked wards and secure units.[4]
- They are more likely to receive major tranquillisers and intramuscular medication and less likely to have counselling or other 'talking treatments'.[5]
- Experiences of racism within mental health services compound their experiences of racism in wider society, for example being stereotyped as unpredictable and violent and being treated with brutality.[6]
- Within our black communities there is a real fear of mental health services – fear of never getting back to ordinary life and even fear of dying as a result of involvement with services.[1]

In his book describing how he and his partners came from the Caribbean and established Britain's biggest black-owned company, Dyke and Dryden Ltd in Tottenham, Tony Wade pointed to other problems in relation to employment.[7]

- Lack of access to capital.
- Few opportunities for black people to experience managerial positions due to the failure of employers to promote them, despite their having the qualifications required.
- Black communities having weak political leverage.

These are the same problems that face black people today. Although we talk about new ways of doing things, we are hampered by the old governing principles that are still in place. Many people talk about the issues to do with black people and work but because they do not know enough about the history, their provision is often reactive and piecemeal.

So why do young black men face these problems? In my experience, low expectations in the education system are where much of the responsibility lies. In school I was put in a special needs class but in the notes from one of my Mental Health Act tribunals, the doctor wrote that I have an IQ above average. Some contradiction! A black professional friend told me that a careers advisor said that he should become a veterinary surgeon's assistant. After pressing them for more information he found that the job entailed mostly cleaning out animals' cages. The more I talk to people, the more of these stories I hear.

Low expectations in the mental health system contribute too, as does the benefits system. Mental health services are based on fear instead of potential and the new Mental Health Bill plays to that same tune. High dosages of medication mean that many people will not move into work because the side effects make them unable to stand being in any kind of work environment. And the complicated benefits system means that once you have completed the mountain of complex forms, you will think twice about coming away from it, just in case you need to complete them all over again if you need the help.

As for the effects, Dr Myles Munroe[8] said that the wealthiest spot on the planet is not the oil fields of Kuwait, Iraq or Saudi Arabia. Neither is it the gold and diamond mines of South Africa, the uranium mines of the Soviet Union or the silver mines of Africa. Though it may surprise you, the richest deposits on our planet lie just a few blocks from your house. They rest in your local cemetery or graveyard. Buried beneath the soil within the walls of those sacred grounds are dreams that never came to pass, songs that were not sung, books that were never written, paintings that never filled a canvas, visions that never became reality.

## Establishing Unlocking Potential in London

Designing marketing material and therefore building a strong identity was important for establishing Unlocking Potential in London, in order to give it street credibility. Service providers were impressed with our logo and everything that was mailed out to them had the invisible word 'professionalism' written all over it. One of the proudest moments was to see Hackney Social Services' logo alongside our own on our materials. Another important part of the process was to create partnerships with as many people and organisations in East London as we could. We formed a steering group with people from Kush Housing Association, Refugee Employment and Mentoring Project, City Hackney Mind, Hackney Social Services and the Disability Employment Advisors at JobCentre Plus. With all of these key players on board, we were able to tap local intelligence and facilitate the achievement of people's dreams. We also mapped out the area of East London and developed a directory, which made things easier when linking people to their desired goals.

## The model

Unlocking Potential London implemented a model of listening, learning and linking (Figure 11.1).

- We listened to the men's dreams.
- We learned how we could best help them.
- We linked them to training or employment services.

Just by asking the men the right questions and actively listening, I could learn about what they really wanted to do. I would ask them 'What is your dream?'

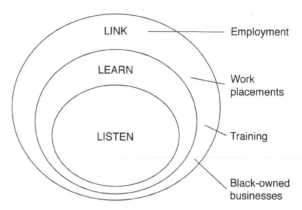

**Figure 11.1:** The Unlocking Potential model.

or perhaps 'What did you like doing when you were younger?'. Together we would develop a strategy for how to get to where they wanted to be and the first step was often by linking them to a training provider. During the year I was involved, Unlocking Potential in London engaged 17 men altogether, helping one into work and about seven into training.

## My own role

As well as offering inspiration, hope, coping strategies and general support, I also aimed to give the men relevant information about their options and to facilitate their access to services. The fact that I had been in the mental health system meant that I was able to understand some of their main concerns. I believe that everyone was born to fulfil a specific purpose and this belief came out in the way that I communicated with the men. I would call them winners, explaining that out of approximately 900 000 sperm, you were the only one that made it alive. I told them that they were here for a purpose and that the world would be a poorer place without them.

Words like these raise the level of expectation and hope in the minds of the men and if hope really ignites, then we move into the area of possibilities. It is all about shifting their state of mind from receiving negative thoughts to positive ones. It is also about encouraging people to market their skills. For instance, someone might mention that they have the gift of writing poems and the question from service providers should then be 'How can we help you use this gift for a living?'. That person could go into copy writing, updating information on websites, writing for magazines, they could go on a creative writing course. It isn't that difficult to explore how someone's area of interest could be turned into business ideas. But many service providers would not see writing as a suitable career, and would probably say something like 'Can you contribute a poem to our newsletter?'.

The lack of insight into how to identify an individual's potential among social workers, psychiatrists and JobCentre Plus workers means that people's dreams are often left untapped and never even encouraged. I have had interviews and yes, they would ask me about the gap in my curriculum vitae. I would just say that I was stressed for a while but I do not spend too much time discussing it. I may have also told them that I was studying and any other thing that would have promoted my application. After all, I was not there to tell them what I wasn't doing, I was there to sell my skills to them and show how I could profit their business.

We also started Hope in a Vessel, which was a tool of encouragement to the men. I used greeting cards with heartening words in them that were relevant to their current situations. I received a brilliant call from a guy that I sent a card to. He had an examination to sit and he stated that the card that I sent to him was instrumental in giving him the right mindset to sit the exam and pass it. The card had a picture of Muhammad Ali standing over Sonny Liston on it and inside I wrote these words, 'You can conquer anything'. He told me that he read those words over and over again as he approached the examination room and out of 10 people who sat the exam, he was the only one to pass it.

## A case study

Every Thursday I attended a day service and met up with the men there on an informal basis. I was introduced to a young man who was 25 years old. At first it seemed that he did not have much to say but after a few weeks he began to open up. Because of the negative experiences that he had been through, his expectation level was very low. Whenever I asked him what his dream was, he would come out with menial jobs. As the mutual respect grew, he started to become more ambitious. I listened carefully to him talking about computers and was able to draw up a simple action plan and research what I learned from our conversation. The next time that we met I told him about the Learn Direct computer training course (www.learndirect.co.uk). He wanted to go ahead with it, so we booked him in for an induction and follow-up sessions. He did not have a personal computer, so we managed to get him a second-hand one. He has now got a qualification in computing and is attending mainstream college. As he says, 'I knew what I wanted to do but I did not have the confidence or know-how to do it. Unlocking Potential helped me through the maze'.

## What worked well?

As Graham said in the last chapter, a central idea behind the Unlocking Potential initiative was that the two projects should develop in line with the needs of local service users. Originally, we thought that the London project would use group work like the project in Sheffield but I found that working one to one with the men enabled me to make far more progress than when I worked with them in groups. Support groups which involve some sharing of emotional needs through discussion are not what the men wanted. Also, many young men are not willing to identify themselves as people with mental health problems and wish above all to integrate within society as ordinary citizens, so a formal 'self-help' group for mental health service users is not useful.

Being able to meet the men in their own homes or over lunch or a game of pool made it possible for them to relax and consequently open up. We were very flexible with the men. Phone calls made in the evening or weekends were always much appreciated, because when you think about it, it is a long time from Friday evening to Monday morning. We determined not to make Unlocking Potential too prescriptive. Learn Direct was a great resource and one that we linked more men to than anywhere else. This was because there was no referral system and the staff did not have to know about people's medical history. The men could also complete the course at their own pace and they were treated like anyone else attending courses. As one put it: 'Learn Direct is like my new day care service'.

We found that building relationships with the men's families enabled us to support the men better. This seemed to be because families often did not understand what their loved ones were going through and to meet someone who had actually come through the system gave them new hope. I believe that families and communities are the best resource for achieving the healing support that we require.

Developing simple action plans was very useful for the men to see their own progress and for us to evaluate what we were achieving. Trying to keep the men focused on their futures helped a lot, because some of them had very unpleasant pasts. It is impossible to change the past but by doing something about our today, our future dreams and plans become obtainable. I threw out small, achievable challenges to the men regularly. I told one man to buy a gardening magazine over the weekend, because that was his area of interest. Immediately he had a goal, something that *he* could do to invest in himself and his future. I have learned that what you keep saying, you eventually believe in and can develop the confidence to achieve.

## What didn't work so well?

Not being able to link the men to relevant agencies quickly enough was a major stumbling block, especially as the men's confidence was built up and there was a real risk of this being hampered. We had to deal with the common problem of organisations not getting back to us. Another problem was the lack of flexibility in the training resources available. One guy wanted to do a course in shoe making but we could not access the resources for him to do this. The unique nature of the course meant the cost was substantial and we could not find funding for it.

The low expectations of service providers were evident in the kind of training that *was* readily on offer. Some of the rubbish initiatives I heard about would not even prepare a fish for water. What needs to be recognised is the entrepreneurial spirit in the black communities. Research in 2003 by the Global Entrepreneurship Monitor shows that most new business start-ups come from black and minority ethnic communities ([www.emkf.org](www.emkf.org)). But for far too long the mental health system has not understood this, often labelling people's ideas as 'grandiose', as was stated in my own medical notes.

The lack of support when the men actually got into work was stark. Some people think that getting a job will solve all their problems and consequently a lot of effort is put into achieving that goal. However, when they get there they soon realise that there are a whole host of new skills that are needed in order to maintain a job. We had a case where employers did not plan for the kind of support that one of our men needed and unfortunately he had a relapse.

Working with black businesses, as shown in Figure 11.1, should have been a very useful tool but there were not enough businesses available to link people to. This was because a lot of black businesses do not have the infrastructure needed to take on trainees or employees. One idea I had, when I walked into a training suite with brand new computers and no one using them, was that these resources could be provided to small businesses to enable them to take on trainees. A 'floating' human resources centre, which could meet the needs of these businesses by providing them with information on employment law, insurance, education, etc. is another idea.

## Conclusion

There is a feasible alternative to what mental health services currently do. Allow me a moment to dream, will you? Someone has to make use of mental health services, so information about their employment and training goals is logged onto a database. Maybe it is called a personal development plan. This would be their roadmap to success and storing the information on a computer database would mean that it would not get lost with changes of staff and could be updated when the service user wanted. This sort of system is used by other successful industries, so why not? Relevant courses would also be available on the wards, so that people have qualifications on their CV, not a massive gap. While in hospital some people could be studying for an Open University degree, if the support to achieve their potential was there.

Being economically independent has given me the confidence to buy my own home and to have holidays, because I do not have to notify the benefits agency when I go away. But most of all, I feel proud to be able to contribute my skills and talents for the betterment of the community. The motto of Unlocking Potential in London was 'Developing You to Develop Your Community'. The mental health system will only become a success when its users feel that entering it is not a destination but a stage to pass through while working towards their purpose by identifying their potential and when the system has the resources to support the release of that potential. I believe that the greatest thing that all concerned about people's fulfilment in work can offer is hope. The person who says 'You can do it' and 'We will do all we can to see you manifest your dreams', and actually does what they say, is the real hero.

Hope is the fuel for the dream. Hope is the strength of the dream. Hope is the incubator that keeps the dream strong in troubled times. Hope is the highest mountain, as we skydive to meet destiny, its physical reality.

## References

1 Sainsbury Centre for Mental Health (2002) *Breaking the Circles of Fear: a review of the relationship between mental health services and African and Caribbean communities.* Sainsbury Centre for Mental Health, London.
2 Bhugra D, Leff J, Mallett R *et al.* (1997) Incidence and outcome of schizophrenia in Whites, African-Caribbeans and Asians in London. *Psychological Medicine.* **27**: 791–8.

3 Bean P, Bingley W, Bynoe I *et al.* (1991) *Out of Harm's Way*. MIND, London.

4 Bolton P (1984) Management of compulsorily admitted patients to a high security unit. *International Journal of Social Psychiatry*. **30**: 77–84.

5 Littlewood R and Cross S (1980) Ethnic minorities and psychiatric services. *Sociology of Health and Illness*. **2**(2): 194–201.

6 Secker J and Harding C (2002) African and African Caribbean users' perceptions of in-patient services. *Journal of Psychiatric and Mental Health Nursing*. **9**(2): 161–8.

7 Wade T (2001) *How They Made a Million: the Dyke and Dryden story*. England Hansib Publications, London.

8 Munroe M 2002 *Understanding your Potential*. Nassau Bahamas Destiny Image Publishers, Nassau.

# Chapter 12

# What's worked for us?

John Marshall, Jo Shenton and Richard Watts

## Introduction

We were asked to write this chapter because we all have experience of supported employment at Rethink Graphics in Brentwood, Essex. Rethink Graphics is a design and print business that is also part of Rethink Employment and Training. The staff work in the recovery model, aiming to increase people's skills, confidence and career options through creative and administrative team work when they are referred, usually by the local CMHT.

As for us, John has been an employment coordinator at Rethink Graphics for six years, before which he was a service user. He also has a part-time business as a wedding and portrait photographer and has just purchased his own shop premises, which will enable him to move on from Rethink in a year or so, becoming full-time self-employed. Jo was a client of the project and now works there part-time, assisting in training and support work as well as shop and design work. She is also self-employed as an Indian head massage therapist and is becoming a well-known local artist, with several exhibitions under her belt. Richard is being supported by the project to achieve his ambition of earning his living through freelance writing – but he will tell you more about that. We'll let John kick off, not because he's the coordinator but because he's first alphabetically. Sticking to that order of things, Jo will then tell you her story so far. Last but only alphabetically, Richard will describe his adventures in employment to date.

## John's perspective

I am a great believer in empowering people to think and decide for themselves, and to be fully aware of the reasons for their choices. I would like to share with you my view on how people can be helped back to work. The dictionary tells me that the verb 'to employ' means 'to make use of the services of a person'. That's apt because everyone needs to feel useful – it's human nature. If you feel useful in the work you do and get on OK with the people you work with, you're likely to be pretty happy in your job. When you don't feel useful and don't get on with the people at work, you can get stressed. They are the two most common reasons I hear for people leaving their job through mental ill health.

But there's more to it than that. People have private lives as well, they may have traumas going on at home or their journey to work could be a trauma in itself. When you add those private problems to any problems at work, then that person is going to suffer.

So what happens when someone who has experienced a mental illness wants to return to work? Assuming the person feels ready to begin their progress towards employment, it is vital that those involved in helping them with that progress get it right and use the right approach. Number one is that the person needs help exploring their options. Unfortunately, many professionals and agencies get this wrong. It's frightening to hear professionals who still assume a client should be limited to performing mundane tasks or that they should simply return to the job they used to do before they were ill, disregarding the person's reluctance to return to that job. More worrying is that many professionals take over and assume they will need to get that person a job, rather than believing they could be assisted to get their own job. To help someone explore their employment options, you need to help them investigate what is good for them, what *they* want to do – and why.

It is vital to keep asking why. This helps the employment worker and client keep things specific when coming to conclusions and the person seeking assistance needs specific conclusions to help them choose what is best for them.

One of the most common issues for people when returning to work after a period of mental ill health is not knowing what they want to do – long term or short term. When this is the case, an approach I have found works well is to ask the client what they would *like* to do, assuming they had the relevant qualifications and so on. Even if what they would like to do turns out to be unsuitable, you can still learn about the different aspects of the job that interested them. With this information you can then help them get the necessary skills to do the job they would like, identify a job that has similar aspects or use the information as part of the bigger picture you are building in search of an alternative job that suits them. We need to start from what the client's realistic wishes are and then seek that opportunity out.

Another important aspect to explore is to find out why any previous employment was so stressful – it's unlikely just to be the actual tasks involved in the job that caused problems. Was it their colleagues? If so, in what way? Was it the actual tasks of the job? If so, narrow down which tasks and why. Was it private problems combined with work? Was it the environment – was it too frantic or too quiet? If you don't know why your client hated working in a shop, for example, then you may go along with them in ignoring shop work as an option for the future, when a job in a different shop might be ideal. However, if you knew that in that job they had a particularly vindictive boss, unrealistic sales targets to meet and a journey Phileas Fogg would struggle with, then you would have a better picture of the real issues.

Before rejecting a certain type of work as an option, we need to be sure exactly why; not all shops are sales-driven, not all offices are hectic or dull, not all colleagues and customers are unpleasant.

When someone already knows the kind of work they would like or has been helped to decide this, a good approach is to map out a path towards what the client wants to achieve and then work through the various obstacles and solutions along the way. In doing this, everyone can keep the goal clearly in view and become clear about what is required to achieve it.

In addition to helping the client identify options that suit them and map out the path towards their goal, it's vital to monitor progress and encourage new challenges and new successes. Even when achieving their goal is going to involve very gradual progress, that path still needs to be designed with the individual in mind and achievements along the way recognised.

If voluntary work is part of the client's pathway, the same care should be taken to make sure the job is suitable as with paid work. Ask what the client is going to get out of it and how it will help them on their way.

I'm not naïve enough to think that everyone can get a job they totally enjoy but I'm experienced enough to know that we all need to enjoy a good proportion of our working day to stay motivated. There will always be aspects to work that aren't ideal – that's life. But mental illness or not, anyone choosing a new career needs to focus on what their passion is and be prepared to take some risks on the way. I love quotes so I will end with one:

> A ship is safe in the harbour but that isn't what it's made for.

## Jo's story so far

I am the oldest of three children. From the age of 14 I have been ill, on and off over the years. I was admitted to hospital for 22 weeks with anorexia nervosa when I was 14, two weeks into starting my third year at senior school. I had always watched my weight; it was a combination of picking up on family problems and the pressure I felt from the media and my peer group. If I overheard someone making negative comments about someone's weight, I would automatically think that they were talking about me and then cut down on my eating. My way of coping with any problems I had was just to either stop eating or cut down my food intake. In my mind that was how I could control a situation or at least feel as if I was able to. Looking back now after coming through several years of therapy, I can see that it was a way of punishing myself too. If I was hurting myself, then I thought, no one else could get hurt.

Once I was released from hospital I carried on with psychotherapy and had home tuition for three years, managing to attain six GCSEs with just two hours' tuition a day. I couldn't bear the thought of going to school and can remember begging my mum not to send me back into school each evening. The fear I felt around people and the bullying I took was just too much for me to cope with. I would rather die, so slowly I tried to, by not eating. When I was admitted to hospital I was told that if I carried on the way I did I would be dead in two weeks. I can remember my mum crying and me just thinking, blimey I've nearly done it. Anorexia had become my closest friend and my worst enemy, taking over my life.

It was whilst I was slowly starving myself that I first began to have hallucinations. It was always a male figure just waiting to get me and telling me to do things that I didn't want to do, like hurt my family. I was told I was seeing these things because I was starving my brain.

I started to cut myself early on too, when I felt angry with someone else or myself. It was a way of releasing any pain I felt and the guilt I felt for feeling angry with someone else. Instead of voicing my feelings, I kept them in so as not to upset anyone and, as a perfectionist, to try to keep up my wanna-be-perfect image. I was brought up a Catholic and in some ways I had convinced myself that it was OK to hurt myself but not other people, treat others the way you would like to be treated, and I carried a lot of guilt over the years, about my illness and how I had nearly destroyed my family and what I had put them all through.

I was OK for several years, though, on and off. I went to art college, something I'd always wanted to do, and then I discovered cannabis! Well, you do when you're at college, and even that was OK too. I was known for my joints and my beetle bong car and I was always popular. After a year at the university doing printed textiles, I was involved in an accident during the summer and decided to take a year out. During that year I went to India and discovered that I wanted to join the university of life. I never went back to art college. One day I might go back but then I was happy and in love. Even so, my mental health problems were always on the back burner simmering away, waiting to explode, and that's what they did.

Around the end of 2001 things came to a head, my head! I lost my job because I wanted to party over the Christmas period and things slowly got worse. I was living in Hove just outside Brighton at the time and it was great living by the sea but everything was to excess. I had started drinking a lot on a regular basis and was smoking a lot too. It reached a point where I was afraid every minute of every day. I was scared and paranoid; boy, was I paranoid. I couldn't read a book, a newspaper, a letter, anything without thinking that there were hidden messages for me to understand. Every time I went outside, I could hear people talking about me, plotting against me. Even in my own flat I thought that my so-called friends and boyfriend at the time were trying to poison me. I wanted to hurt them and my closest family. I was absolutely convinced that there was some kind of conspiracy against me and there was no way of seeing an end to it. Part of me just wanted it all over, to die, but there was a small part of me that didn't want to give in and let 'them' get their way, with me out of the way.

I went to the doctor and over the next couple of months I was treated with drugs for depression and anxiety with psychotic episodes. This basically meant I was put into a state of numbness, staring into space and at times dribbling; basically I was a vegetable, unable to talk. It felt like my mind was paralysed, unable to do anything apart from rest. In a way it was a relief and probably what I needed at the time. I slept so much but my mind and body needed to sleep. I used to be afraid of falling asleep because then I would dream and my dreams were scary.

Eventually I was admitted to a psychiatric ward for two weeks. I don't really remember much about it, apart from feeling that I had finally hit a really low point in my life and that maybe I was in the right place after all now, this was going to be it for me, the end. Always the drama queen. But it wasn't the end at all.

My social worker from the CMHT suggested that I might be able to come to Rethink Graphics, to break up my day, give me some purpose to getting up in the morning and learn some computer skills. Once I started there, attending a two-hour training slot once a week, I built up my confidence on the computer and took and passed my Computer Literacy And Information Technology (CLAIT) exams, which in turn built up my confidence some more. I gave myself a chance to make mistakes and learn from them and started to get some structure back into my life that didn't revolve around just being ill. Even just making tea for people in the shop was good for me. I was helping out and made to feel welcome and that I had a place there.

Rethink has been a positive part in my life. When I started, my self-esteem was low and I didn't talk to many people, mainly because I was just scared sometimes. I've learnt how to interact with people without being so scared that I'm going to be judged. I wasn't laughed at either about the worries I had going around in my head and I was respected as an individual. A little later on I started working in the shop, serving customers and learning the ropes of how the shop works and the printing side of Rethink Graphics. I learnt that I was a valued person and that my skills were skills that were useful and could help people.

I was given help and support to claim the benefits I was entitled to whilst I was ill and once I started part-time work, I was advised which benefits I was eligible for. Without Rethink Graphics, I think my life could have gone a different way, it might have taken me longer to get to recovery.

Recovery is the key word at Rethink Graphics. I was encouraged and valued whenever I attended and gradually I learnt that I wasn't alone in my thoughts, like I thought I was. What do you mean, you're paranoid too? If everyone's out to get me, how can they have time to get you too? After all, the whole world revolves around me-me-me, not you-you-you! This is quite a comforting thought, along with my sense of humour that keeps me going. At least today I am able to laugh again and I feel a long way off from the scared paranoid child I once was. It's still easy for my mind to run away with ideas if I let it but that's the key – if I let it. I have a choice now. I've always had choices but now I choose to listen to my body and my head. I know the warning signs. If I'm in a low patch, I could easily spiral down again. But if I talk about what's happening for me, and hear myself talking about it, it helps to put things in perspective and realise that I'm not alone. There isn't anything I can't do today if I set my mind to it. My life is for living so I just get on and live.

Thanks for your eyes.

## Richard's employment adventures to date

Perhaps in contrast to the general emphasis of this book, employment has been a bogey word for me since I left university. I had a series of very early psychotic episodes as a pre-teen and adolescent, so it was a miracle that I reached university at all and I was very grateful to get there. Despite three hospitalisations between the ages of 14 and 16, and a reluctant diagnosis of schizoaffective disorder being made, I went on to complete three A Levels and to gain a good degree at Reading University. During periods of illness, I suffered from all the symptoms of schizophrenia as well as intense mood swings and after my third time in hospital, I continued to take antipsychotic, mood-stabilising and anti-depressant medication.

Despite this, I had what I consider my hiatus from mental illness between the ages of 17 and about 23 and was able to complete my education. There was a sense of comfortable complacency leading up to graduation that things had been going smoothly and would continue in the same way. On leaving Reading, I began a course in newspaper journalism because I had enjoyed my English degree and writing for the student newspaper. This is when my problems in coping began to reoccur. I was living at home again and getting a bus to college and my work placement at a newspaper.

The course was intensely competitive. The tutors fostered a kind of rivalry between the students which didn't suit me, especially since I fell behind in the important aspect of shorthand and never really caught up. It was also a short and intensive course with a clear pass-or-fail on every exam and no real chance to right mistakes. Towards the end I had a terrible sense of wanting to leave the course and I begged my parents to let me but they were paying for the course and persuaded me to see it through.

As the course ended with exam results pending, I had an apparent reversal of fortune when I gained a job on a local newspaper in Berkshire. I went back to Reading and rented a room while I began my traineeship. There were a few anxieties, like my problems with shorthand, which was a requirement and yet I hadn't mastered it. I began to have fallings-out with a few contacts, in particular a local councillor who accused me of writing an inaccurate article about him, despite his inability to remember what it was about. I later suspected he had confused me with a former trainee whom I replaced but at the time it was a real blow to my confidence and I imagined word would get around not to talk to 'that shoddy young reporter'.

Without anyone at home to support me, events speeded up and I voiced my concerns about the job to my news editor. These were interpreted as more or less my desire to leave, rather than a request for a supporting word. It was only my fifth week in the job and day after day I felt more desperate and unable to carry on the work. I felt extremely isolated in the office. All the other staff bar the editor and one advertising agent were female and this somehow added to my sense of alienation. After a talk in the editor's office, I left the job and came home to my parents the same week.

Over the next few months I claimed jobseekers' allowance and tried to get another job doing some sort of journalism or another interesting job, perhaps in the arts field as I loved literature and music in particular. Eventually this led me to take a job in a music shop in East London. It was a complete change to the newspaper, very quiet a lot of the time with some quite childish banter and leg-pulling from the other two shop assistants, who were both bored in the job. I was determined not to have a repeat of my first job and stayed there, learning the 'knowledge' of selling and hiring out musical instruments and the intricacies of the shop. Unfortunately, the managing director of the firm told us one afternoon he would have to shut the branch because it wasn't viable and because the manager was leaving and couldn't be replaced.

Next I worked for another music shop in the West End of London. This seemed good at first, like the newspaper, but after a month my grandad died suddenly and that threw my mental health out of balance. I felt sick at work, vomited and had to go home a few times. Eventually I quit, feeling really defeated. I worked for my local Marks & Spencer over Christmas, where the work was mindless but at least it was busy and lively among the younger staff.

The next year, 2001, I got a job at a local bookshop but I was just putting books out all day. It left me feeling frustrated and sure I could do better and I began to get a sense of injustice about the world of work. Within a year my work prospects seemed to have gone from having a graduate-level trainee journalism career to being a shop assistant and there appeared to be no way back.

The next couple of years were desperate times during which I repeatedly began new ventures only to find them unbearably tedious and/or had fallings-out with staff members or the boss. I did a few temping jobs in offices, which were far from ideal because they were so uncertain and often finished just as I was getting used to them. In job after job I also suffered from the paranoid belief that people were talking about me and singling me out for harsh treatment and my behaviour would deteriorate as a result. Often, the worse I felt, the less work I did and I was sacked from several jobs. It reminded me of being scapegoated at school and sent out of classrooms when everyone had been messing about.

The burden of not having a 'proper' job became everything to me and was exacerbated by the countless 'well wishers' and acquaintances who always asked me 'What are you doing?'. I wasn't sure what made me feel worse, the lack of personal satisfaction or the constant reminders of it from other people. I failed to attribute my employment problems to my mental health, which put the burden onto my lack of ingenuity and lack of hard grind. I decided there had to be another way of escaping this 'employment trap' of menial shop and office work.

I was doing some creative writing so I tried to get onto an MA in creative writing. As a fallback I applied for a regular English MA. The creative writing course rejected me but the English one accepted me, so I looked forward to returning to studying. I hoped to do the academic thing, follow up the MA with a PhD and become a university lecturer, although perhaps it was too ambitious. The pressure I'd put on myself to excel became too much even before the course started and that year I didn't begin it. I also stopped taking my antidepressants, becoming obsessed with the inhibiting effects of all my medication on my mental functioning.

The result was that I became extremely unmotivated and depressed and spent nearly a whole year unemployed. It was a bleak time that was only countered by some helpful counselling I received through Mind. Following advice, I retook my driving test and passed it third time, which boosted my confidence even if nothing else did. I was also referred to an NHS psychiatrist for the purpose of being put on a more modern antipsychotic (I had been seeing a doctor privately for a long time and he didn't know much about new medications). At the same time I re-enrolled on my MA and started it in 2002. Once again there were problems, this time from the tiredness due to the new drug, which turned out to be quite an old one! I quit the course after my trademark one month and did voluntary work at a charity shop.

Meanwhile I was referred to Rethink Graphics and talked to their employment advisor. Having abandoned the grandiose aim of being a lecturer, I was left with nothing to aim at. I did get paid work at the charity shop and was put on better medication, although it gave me headaches that wouldn't go away, but my job was a temporary post. When I heard that it was finishing, I began to go off the rails. I was losing a lot of weight and there were lots of arguments with people at work and with my parents at home but all the time I was getting increasingly enthusiastic about the idea that I would be healed. I am a Christian and had recently started going to a Pentecostal church where such things as healing and spiritual gifts were not only talked about but practised. Perhaps I was becoming a religious maniac.

One Sunday night I believed I had received my healing during the service and a few weeks later, soon after my job finished, I stopped taking my medication, to 'test it'. I don't think I would have stopped my medication if I were still working. My life had become very empty without work, after coping with a job for a period of time for the first time in my life, and thoughts of healing replaced it.

In summer 2003 I was hospitalised and was very ill, much worse than my previous episodes as a teenager. I was discharged from hospital in late October. Since then I have not worked and have attended Rethink Graphics twice a week. The staff had already helped me to hold down my charity shop job until it ended. If I was having a bad day, I'd ring the employment advisor and if things couldn't be resolved on the phone, he'd meet me for lunch and talk over my concerns. On reflection, the problems were mostly from hostile or misinterpreted comments from the elderly volunteers and he helped me to see them in a clearer perspective.

Over the last nine months I've attended Rethink Graphics regularly and the team there have provided sympathetic support for my mental ups and downs, talking over my daily struggles and progress in a way that has helped me see where I stand. It's been hard to judge my overall mental health on my own while I've been recovering from last summer's illness, other than constantly thinking how exhausted I am and thinking I'm not doing enough. People at Rethink have helped me to see I've been improving and given me feedback on fluctuations that I wouldn't notice alone.

They've also followed the 'recovery model', consistently aiming to motivate me into doing small work projects, and the consistency has meant that when I have felt better I've been able to achieve more than I'd have hoped. In particular, I've contributed to the Rethink Graphics newsletter, almost writing half of it at times, and this has been built up until jointly we've come up with the idea of my becoming a paid freelance writer. Here again they have helped me by finding work for me and continuing to provide a momentum for my progress. It's not like previous ambitions that haven't come to fruition because I've lost my confidence before they started. The team at Rethink provide a tangible means of keeping the idea of writing buoyant from week to week. This would be difficult on my own, especially in weeks when nothing has been achieved.

With the support of the staff and my parents, I have decided not to repeat my attempts to hold down regular work but to take a different approach. I am now starting to work as a freelance writer and with the help of the Rethink staff and their contacts, I have already obtained three paid commissions for written work, including the current piece.

Sometimes it seems like an excuse not to 'work' in the usual sense but my new venture is still in its initial stages and I have convinced myself to be patient. I believe I could become a professional writer. Lots of people compliment me on my writing skills and I am positive that at last I have settled on a worthwhile and, dare I say it, realistic solution to my employment problems. It's better to take a small step at a time with the support of other people than to set yourself a massive target. We can't ignore our previous failings but neither can we give up.

# Part 3

# Avoiding the slippery slope

# Chapter 13

# Getting off the slippery slope: what do we know about what works?

Tina Thomas and Jenny Secker

## Introduction

If you are working and begin to experience mental health problems, what are your chances of keeping your job? A survey carried out in a psychiatric hospital in the city of Bristol[1] aimed to answer that question by finding out how many of the 60 service users in hospital on the day of the survey had lost their job as a result of experiencing mental health problems. Forty-five (75%) of the 60 service users agreed to be interviewed and 35 (78%) of them reported having lost one or more jobs as a result of their mental ill health. The main reasons for people sliding down the slippery slope towards unemployment and being unable to extricate themselves revolved around a complete lack of focus within mental health services on supporting people in work to keep their job when they came into contact with services.

The survey results gave impetus to the development of a job retention service within the Avon and Wiltshire Mental Health Partnership NHS Trust. The Department of Health and the Department for Work and Pensions provided assistance with funding and also commissioned an evaluation of the service (*see* Chapter 14 for an account of the evaluation). In order to inform both the development of the service and the evaluation, we carried out a review of the international literature to see what could be learnt from experience elsewhere about getting people off the slippery slope before they have slid too far down.

The review revealed two relevant areas of research: studies examining the barriers to job retention and research into what works in improving job retention rates.

## Barriers to job retention

Much of the evidence relating to barriers to job retention derives from research with people returning to the labour market after experiencing mental ill health rather than with those already in jobs. A few studies have, however, focused on this group and evidence from research with both populations indicates that the major barriers to job retention revolve around three issues: employers discriminating against people with mental health problems; an associated reluctance to disclose problems and use the support available, compounded by lack of awareness of employment rights; and low expectations among both mental health professionals and those experiencing mental health problems.

## Discrimination

Studies have found that people experiencing mental health problems are likely to encounter discrimination on the part of employers and managers. Employees with mental health problems report discriminatory attitudes and practices among employers, with between a third and a half of study participants indicating that they had been dismissed, 'forced to resign', redeployed or made redundant because of discrimination.[2,3] Among a sample of 43 people on sick leave with mental health problems, Gates reported that almost half thought it likely that they would lose their job because of their condition.[4] Even if job loss does not result, employees report reduced opportunities for advancement[5] and managers have indeed been shown to view employees with mental health problems as incapable of taking on new challenges.[6]

## Reluctance to disclose and take up support

Closely related to discriminatory attitudes, reluctance to disclose a mental health problem to an employer or manager creates a further barrier to job retention in that this can clearly impact on take-up of the entitlement to reasonable work adjustments under both the UK Disability Discrimination Act (DDA) of 1995 and the American Disabilities Act (ADA) of 1990. Moreover, if a person with a mental health problem is dismissed from their job for poor performance and had not disclosed their mental health problem to their employer, then these legal frameworks afford them no protection.[7] In a North American study of employees with a mental illness, Granger found many were concerned that their employers would misuse information about their illness by either talking about them to other employees or judging their work performance on their disability rather than their productivity.[5] Some employees lost their jobs or chose to resign rather than disclose their illness. However, lack of awareness of entitlement to adjustments was also found to be a significant barrier as 86% of participants were unfamiliar with the ADA. Similarly, Blackwell *et al.* report poor awareness among UK employees concerning the inclusion of mental illness in the DDA.[6]

Failure to take up workplace adjustments and other types of support is also relevant where problems on the job are concerned. A recent study of 84 clients from a supported employment programme who had gained at least one job found that 75% experienced job termination within 18 months, with an average length of employment of only 13 weeks.[8] When satisfactory terminations (e.g. left for another job or left because the job was time limited) were compared with unsatisfactory terminations (e.g. fired or left without another job), symptoms, diagnosis, initial job satisfaction and initial perceived working environment were not found to be related to type of termination. However, reported problems on the job did discriminate between the two groups. Those who had unsatisfactory job terminations, and their employers, reported more interpersonal problems, greater job dissatisfaction, poorer work quality and more medical-related problems than people who had satisfactory terminations. The authors concluded that unsatisfactory job terminations are largely due to adverse reactions and events that occur once a competitive job is in progress.

## Low expectations

Users of mental health services report that the expectations of mental health professionals regarding their vocational potential are very low and that work is regarded by professionals as an unrealistic goal.[9-11] These perceptions are confirmed by clinicians themselves, who report finding it difficult to believe that clients can maintain jobs and who also express concerns about the potential consequences of employment failure on their clients' mental health.[12] Thus clinicians often do not even enquire whether newly referred clients are employed and the issue of job retention is rarely addressed.

In turn, low expectations among mental health professionals are likely to compound service users' own low expectations of themselves. During and following a period of mental ill health, it is not uncommon for a person to experience a decrease in self-esteem, either as a part of the mental illness (e.g. depression) or as a consequence of the stigma attached to it.[13-15] Many people who experience mental health problems underestimate their own capacity to work and internalise the idea of being unemployable, which can lead to decreased confidence in the ability to return to the labour market, further mental health problems and social exclusion.[16,17]

# Factors associated with job retention

Factors that emerge from the literature as likely to promote job retention can be categorised as relating to the individual, the workplace and the relationship between the two.

## Individual factors

At the individual level, Kirsh compared people with a mental illness who had successfully retained employment to those who had not and found no differences between the two groups on any individual factors or demographics, including diagnosis and hospitalisation history.[18] However, the individual's attitude to their illness and employment has been found to be significant. People with mental illness who gain and maintain employment tend to have a clear perspective on their illness and the place of their illness within their lives more generally.[19] In contrast, those who gain employment but do not maintain it express less sense of the illness being only one aspect of their identity. In addition, those who maintain employment view work as having a role in the recovery process by improving their self-regard and offering some control over symptoms. Similarly, Schneid and Anderson found that in a sample of 10 employed people diagnosed with a mental illness, insight into their illness and a realistic appraisal of their own capabilities in light of the illness were necessary factors for successful job retention.[20]

Also at the individual level, research into both mental health and other disabilities and workplace injuries indicates that the shorter the length of time off work, the greater the likelihood of job retention. On the one hand, extended periods of sick leave decrease the likelihood of return and foster a detachment from work.[21, 22] On the other hand, over-concern, over-diagnosis, over-treatment and advice to remain off work can promote prolonged disability.[23, 24] These studies suggest that intervention is required within 3–6 months of an employee taking sick leave.

## Workplace factors

Within the workplace, research on the prevention of work-related stress has been extended and applied to dealing with mental health problems in the workplace (for a review of this extensive literature, see Merz *et al.*[25]). Akabas argues that the same factors that provide a healthy and productive workplace for non-disabled employees also ensure job retention for people with mental health problems.[26] The factors highlighted include: promoting worker involvement in the job; fostering peer cohesion; encouraging staff support; promoting autonomy; being goal-oriented; minimising work pressure; offering clear expectations; promoting employee control over the job; emphasising innovation; and affording physical comfort. Akabas further argues that this type of work environment can be therapeutic for people with a mental illness in that it empowers workers, allows them to be flexible in the means by which they achieve their work goals and provides ongoing and consistent support.

However, research on job retention among people with mental illness who gain employment with the support of vocational rehabilitation services indicates that ongoing access to more specific support may also be crucial to success.[27–30] The type of support required is aimed primarily at solving problems that arise on the job, a major barrier to job retention, as was seen above.

In addition, there is some evidence that the social characteristics of the workplace are important for long-term job retention. One approach therefore involves linking employees to existing 'natural supports' in the workplace.[31] Natural supports are people within the workplace who are not disability or mental health service providers. They provide assistance, feedback, contact or companionship to enable people with mental health problems to participate independently in the workplace.[32] Research shows that developing such natural supports is more effective and longer lasting than using an external job coach.[32,33]

Over and above the factors so far considered, however, the factor most strongly associated with successful job retention is the support and active involvement of management, since management involvement is required for the successful implementation of return to work plans, workplace adjustments and workplace supports. Research has shown that without the support of the supervisor or manager, return to work and job retention are jeopardised.[4]

# The relationship between individual and workplace factors

While both individual and workplace factors therefore impact on job retention, recent research suggests that the relationship between the two may be an over-arching factor. In Kirsh's study, for example, both organisational climate and person–environment fit, in terms of the correlation between organisational values and individual preferences for these values, were significantly associated with success in retaining a job.[18] Equally, job retention and job tenure have been found to be closely linked with initial job preference and subsequent job satisfaction, both arguably factors in person–environment fit. More specifically, people with mental illness who are employed in their preferred areas of work retain their positions for longer than those who are not working in their preferred areas.[34,35] Individuals with mental illness who report satisfaction with their jobs also remain in their positions longer and are more likely to retain employment than those who report dissatisfaction with their jobs.[36,37] Unsurprisingly, people are also more satisfied with their jobs when they are working in their preferred field of work.[38]

## Conclusion

Overall, the literature illustrates that three distinct sets of issues need to be addressed in relation to employment and mental health. The first is to address issues for the people who have a mental illness, are unemployed and require support in gaining employment. The second is to address issues for the changing stream of people who are employed and experience mental heath problems at work. These people require support in retaining employment and successfully returning to work. If it becomes necessary for an employee to take sick leave, support needs to be offered within 3–6 months and the earlier the better. The third is to address issues for the entire employed population that are at risk of developing mental health problems. This wider group may benefit from attempts to reduce workplace stress and prevent the onset of mental health problems. All three areas are vital to the effective management of employment and mental health issues.

These three distinct groups and corresponding types of services can be understood in terms of the three levels of prevention as defined in the field of public health (*see* Figure 13.1): primary prevention, secondary prevention and tertiary prevention. Primary prevention strategies seek to eliminate causal factors in the development of problems, which in this case refers to attempts to reduce stress in the workplace. Secondary prevention strategies aim to reduce the severity or duration of disorders and to avoid the development of more serious and disabling conditions, which in this case refers to attempts to facilitate job retention and successful return to work. Lastly, tertiary prevention strategies deal directly with existing chronic conditions and are aimed at rehabilitation, which in this case reflects attempts to enable unemployed people with mental illness to find and keep meaningful work.

Previous research and practice have focused mainly on reducing stress in the workplace and on vocational rehabilitation services for unemployed people with mental illness. There is a large gap in research and practice on mental health and job retention. Yet the system cannot be effective for people with mental health problems unless there is support in both maintaining as well as gaining employment. Additionally, primary prevention strategies are not effective for the entire working population and therefore support is needed for people who do develop mental health problems while working to retain their employment. It seems that this gap is resulting in increasing numbers of people losing employment due to

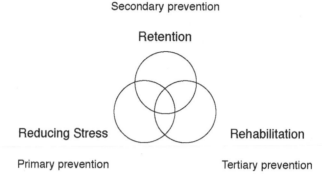

Figure 13.1: **Levels of prevention in relation to three areas of service delivery for mental health and employment.**

mental illness, becoming dependent on welfare benefits and losing a crucial source of self-esteem and self-identity. It is arguable that demand for tertiary prevention services, such as vocational rehabilitation for long-term unemployed people with mental health problems, could be substantially reduced if secondary services, including job retention and return to work interventions, were more widely available to prevent the downward spiral of job loss, detachment from the labour market and decreasing mental health.

When it was established, the Avon and Wiltshire Job Retention Service was the only secondary prevention service in the UK. In Australia, however, the Commonwealth Rehabilitation Service had introduced a case management model aimed at preventing job loss among people from all disability groups[21] and it was on this model that the Avon and Wiltshire service was therefore based. To inform the development of the service, we compared the Australian model with the results of our literature review. Although the model encompassed many of the factors shown in the literature to be important, there were three areas identified by the review that it did not appear to be addressing: the provision of mental health counselling; facilitating natural supports in the workplace; and providing information and advice on employment issues to mental health workers and GPs. By incorporating these with the areas that were addressed by the Australian model, we were able to devise a list of key criteria for effectiveness (Box 13.1) to inform both the development and the evaluation of the Avon and Wiltshire service.

---

**Box 13.1 Key criteria for an effective job retention service**

Vocational counselling – ability to address employment issues, job satisfaction and preference, and disclosure issues without bias and ensuring confidentiality from employer where required by employee

---

Mental health counselling – ability to address mental health issues, symptom management in the workplace, perspectives on illness, psychological detachment from work, self-esteem and self-identity issues, also ensuring confidentiality

Primary allegiance to client

Advocate for client in the workplace

Specialist regarding DDA, legal issues and relevant financial incentives or benefits

Provides training and advice to employers and managers on dealing with mental health issues in the workplace

Provides training to employers on healthy workplaces for all employees

Facilitates communication between employee and employer regarding time off work, return to work plans, modified work programmes and adjustments

Facilitates natural supports within the workplace

Promotes early intervention and is easily accessed by employers and employees

Keeps all parties informed – including employer, employee, mental health workers, GPs

Ongoing support to manage any problems in the workplace as they arise

Provides training and advice on employment issues for people with mental health problems to mental health workers and GPs

# References

1 Butterworth R (2001) Job retention – developing a service. *Mental Health Review.* 6(4): 17–20.
2 Mental Health Foundation (2002) *Out at Work: a survey of the experiences of people with mental health problems within the workplace.* Mental Health Foundation, London.
3 Read J and Baker S (1996) *Not Just Sticks and Stones: a survey of the stigma, taboos and discrimination experienced by people with mental health problems.* Mind, London.
4 Gates L (2000) Workplace accommodation as a social process. *Journal of Occupational Rehabilitation.* 10(1): 85–98.
5 Granger B (2000) The role of psychiatric rehabilitation practitioners in assisting people in understanding how to best assert their ADA rights and arrange job accommodations. *Psychiatric Rehabilitation Journal.* 23(3): 215–23.
6 Blackwell T, Burns P and Hard S (2001) *Working Minds: attitudes on mental health in the workplace, with proposals for change.* The Industrial Society, London.
7 Schneider D (1998) When do I disclose? ADA protection and your job. *Occupational Therapy and Mental Health.* 14(1 and 2): 77–87.
8 Becker D, Drake R, Bond G *et al.* (1998) Job terminations among people with severe mental illness participating in supported employment. *Community Mental Health Journal.* 34(1): 71–82.

9 Read J (1997) What is a good day project? *A Life in the Day.* 1(2): 7–11.

10 Secker J, Grove B and Seebohm P (2001) Challenging barriers to employment, training and education for mental health service users: the service user's perspective. *Journal of Mental Health.* 10(4): 395–404.

11 Webster A (1998) An uncharted journey. *A Life in the Day.* 2(2): 9–12.

12 Harris M, Bebout R, Freeman D *et al.* (1997) Work stories: psychological responses to work in population of dually diagnosed adults. *Psychiatric Quarterly.* 68(2): 131–53.

13 Carrigan P, Watson A (2002) The paradox of self-stigma and mental illness. *Clinical Psychology Science and Practice.* 9(1): 35–53.

14 Costello C (ed.) (1993) *Symptoms of Depression.* John Wiley, New York.

15 Watson D, Suls J and Haig J (2002) Global self-esteem in relation to structural models of personality and affectivity. *Journal of Personality and Social Psychology.* 83(1): 185–97.

16 Duckworth S (2001) The disabled person's perspective. *Report on New Beginnings – A Symposium on Disability.* Unum Limited, Surrey.

17 Garske G and Stewart J (1999) Stigmatic and mythical thinking: barriers to vocational rehabilitation services for persons with severe mental illness. *Journal of Rehabilitation.* 65(4): 4–8.

18 Kirsh B (2000) Factors associated with employment for mental health consumers. *Psychiatric Rehabilitation Journal.* 24(1): 13–21.

19 Cunningham K, Wolbert R and Brockmeier M (2000) Moving beyond the illness: factors contributing to gaining and maintaining employment. *American Journal of Community Psychology.* 29(4): 481–94.

20 Schneid T and Anderson C (1995) Living with chronic mental illness: understanding the role of work. *Community Mental Health Journal.* 31(2): 163–76.

21 BSRM (2001) *Vocational Rehabilitation: the way forward.* British Society of Rehabilitation Medicine, London.

22 Niemeyer L, Jacobs K, Renolds-Llynch K *et al.* (1994) Work hardening: past, present and future – the Work Programs Special Interest Section National Work Hardening Outcome Study. *American Journal of Occupational Therapy.* 48: 327–39.

23 Hall W and Morrow L (1988) Repetition strain injury: an Australian epidemic of upper limb pain. *Social Science and Medicine.* 27: 645–9.

24 Reid J, Ewan C and Lowy E (1991) Pilgrimage of pain: the illness experiences of women with repetition strain injury and the search for credibility. *Social Science and Medicine.* 32: 601–12.

25 Merz M, Bricout J and Koch L (2001) Disability and job stress: implications for vocational rehabilitation planning. *Work.* 17: 85–95.

26 Akabas S (1994) Workplace responsiveness: key employer characteristics in support of job maintenance for people with mental illness. *Psychosocial Rehabilitation Journal.* 17(3): 91–102.

27 Bond G, Drake R, Mueser K *et al.* (1997) An update on supported employment for people with severe mental illness. *Psychiatric Services.* 48(3): 335–44.

28 Chandler D, Meisel J, Hu T *et al.* (1998) A capitated model for cross-section of severely mentally ill clients: employment outcomes. *Community Mental Health Journal.* 34(1): 13–26.

29 McHugo G, Drake R and Becker D (1998) The durability of supported employment effects. *Psychiatric Rehabilitation Journal.* 22: 55–61.

30 Secker J, Membrey H, Grove B *et al.* (2002) Recovering from illness or recovering your life? Implications of clinical versus social models of recovery from mental illness for employment support services. *Disability and Society.* 17(4): 403–18.

31 West M and Parent W (1995) Community and workplace supports for individuals with severe mental illness in supported employment. *Psychosocial Rehabilitation Journal.* 18: 13–24.

32 Storey K and Certo N (1996) Natural supports for increasing integration in the work-

place for people with disabilities: a review of the literature and guidelines for implementation. *Rehabilitation Counseling Bulletin.* **40**(1): 62–76.

33 Fabian E, Waterworth A and Ripke B (1993) Reasonable accommodations for workers with serious mental illnesses: type, frequency and associated outcomes. *Psychosocial Rehabilitation Journal.* **7**(2): 163–72.

34 Becker D, Drake R, Farabaugh A *et al.* (1996) Job preferences of clients with severe psychiatric disorders participating in supported employment programs. *Psychiatric Services.* **47**: 1223–7

35 Freedman R (1996) The meaning of work in the lives of people with significant disabilities: consumer and family perspectives. *Journal of Rehabilitation.* **62**: 49–55.

36 Bond G (1994 Applying psychiatric rehabilitation principles to employment: recent findings. In: R Ancill (ed.) *Schizophrenia: exploring the spectrum of psychosis.* John Wiley, Chichester.

37 Xie H, Dain B, Becker D *et al.* (1997) Job tenure among persons with severe mental illness. *Rehabilitation Counseling Bulletin.* **40**(4): 230–9.

38 Meuser K, Becker D and Wolfe R (2001) Supported employment, job preferences, job tenure, and satisfaction. *Journal of Mental Health.* **10**(4): 411–17.

# Chapter 14

# Getting off the slippery slope: an example from the UK

Tina Thomas and Jenny Secker

## Introduction

As we saw in the previous chapter, the job retention service established by the Avon and Wiltshire Mental Health Partnership Trust was the first service in the UK to focus on secondary prevention; in other words, getting people at risk of losing their jobs as a result of mental health problems off the slippery slope that for too many leads to long-term unemployment. The service is delivered by a job retention team and operates on a case management model based on that developed by the Commonwealth Rehabilitation Service in Australia. Two case managers offer a free service to employees experiencing mental health problems. Referrals to the team come from local GPs.

Funding provided by the Department of Health and the Department for Work and Pensions supported both the development of the project and an evaluation carried out during the first year of its operation. Sixteen clients with whom the job retention team had completed or almost completed work were invited to take part in an interview exploring their views about the service provided and 13 agreed. With the clients' permission, five employers were also interviewed and six GPs took part in a group discussion. The two case managers provided additional information.

In this chapter we first describe the clients and the interventions they received from the job retention team. We then examine the views of the stakeholders we interviewed and the outcomes achieved, concluding by comparing our results with the 13 key effectiveness criteria derived from the international literature and listed in the previous chapter.

## Clients and interventions

All but one of the clients who took part in the evaluation were white, just under two-thirds were female and just over two-thirds were married. Most clients were in their middle years (mean 42 years, range 34–57), with two nearing retirement. Almost all the clients were in full-time employment and had been in their current job for a substantial period of time. The majority had a reasonable level of income commensurate with the employment of three-quarters in managerial or professional roles. Most were employed in medium to large companies. Four clients had severe and enduring mental health problems, while nine had mild to moderate problems, in seven cases a first episode.

Just over half the clients received a service from the job retention team for six months or less, although some continued to receive telephone support as required. Only two were still receiving a service after one year.

The interventions delivered by the team can be categorised as either client focused or work focused. The most common client-focused interventions included supportive counselling, self-esteem building, coping skills and problem-solving development, cognitive behavioural therapy (CBT) and anxiety management. Over half the clients also received support regarding relationship issues. The most common work-focused interventions included mental health awareness raising and education for employers, negotiating workplace adjustments and information or advice on legal issues.

On average, the two case managers reported spending 70% of their time on client-focused interventions (range 50–100%) and 14% of their time on work-focused interventions (range 0–25%). In addition, they spent an average of 4% of their time liaising with other services regarding clients (range 0–30%) and 13% of their time writing letters, making phone calls, organising meetings and writing reports (range 0–20%).

## Perceptions of the service

Stakeholders' perceptions of the job retention service are presented below in relation to:

- the need for a job retention service
- client-focused interventions
- work-focused interventions.

### The need for the service

Across all stakeholder groups there was widespread agreement that a job retention service was needed on four grounds: because work was a significant factor in causing or exacerbating mental health problems; because other services were unable to provide the support required to enable people with mental health problems to stay in work; because employers were not always able to deal effectively with mental health issues; and because early intervention was required to prevent job loss.

Taking the impact of work on mental health first, nine of the 13 clients interviewed for the study believed that work was the major cause of their mental health problems. All four clients who did not believe work to be a major cause of their mental ill health had been living with severe and enduring illness for a number of years. While these clients did not believe that work had directly caused their mental illness, they thought that additional stress at work had a negative impact on their mental health and could trigger symptoms or episodes.

The case managers agreed that for the majority of clients, a stressful work environment was a significant factor, highlighting overwork, poor management, bullying or uncertainty about job role following reorganisations. Addressing these issues with employers was regarded as a key role for the service. More generally, the GPs also thought work was an important factor in the development of mental ill health among their patients and employers too were aware that work had been a causal factor in the development of mental health problems.

> The merger caused a lot of uncertainty and unsettledness and discord. The employee reacted badly to it. I was aware of her personality and discontent and aware of her long-term absenteeism, although I was relatively unfamiliar with the depth of her illness until the last few months. I was also aware that the organisation had not dealt with her well in terms of an organisational change. I had some sympathy for her. (Employer)

Turning to the limitations of other services, for most clients their GP had been their first port of call in seeking help but both they and the GPs themselves agreed that GPs were unable to support them to stay in work. In addition to their GP, three clients had used workplace counselling services or employment assistance programmes (EAPs) provided by their employer, with mixed results from their perspective. While one client had found workplace counselling beneficial, the other two clients reported that the support they had received had not been helpful. Only two clients also mentioned the involvement of their human resources department and neither had found this helpful. As one client commented: 'HR should be about people but often it is only about numbers'.

Mental health services, including community psychiatric nurses (CPNs), a panic clinic and CBT therapists, were mentioned by only a small number of clients, all of whom viewed these services as lacking in expertise regarding work issues.

Where employers' ability to deal with mental health issues was concerned, five clients described treatment at work relating to their mental health problems that they perceived to be unfair or discriminatory. One client who had severe and enduring problems reported being bullied at work and in general clients were concerned by the stigmatisation of mental ill health reflected in the attitudes of some colleagues. For their part, the employers who took part in interviews recognised that attitudes towards mental health in the workplace could be quite negative and acknowledged that they were not trained or provided with the information required to effectively manage employees with mental health problems.

> I think a lot of people are quite uncomfortable in dealing with any kind of mental health or stress issue, they feel a bit unsure of themselves around that. I do think a lot of people don't see them as real illnesses and are afraid to tackle them. (Employer)

Intervening at a sufficiently early stage to prevent job loss is intrinsic to the aims of any job retention service. Since the job retention team was a newly established service, several clients had been experiencing problems at work for some time when they were referred and these clients made clear the need for the earlier intervention others received. Similarly, both the job retention team case managers and the employers spoke of the benefits of early intervention.

> I would say to others to use it sooner rather than later, get involved as soon as you can. They were extremely helpful to me but in a way it was past the point and the damage was done, we never managed to retrieve the situation. (Client)

> There's a need for helping people to get back to work as quickly as possible and not languishing on sickness benefits or in a vacuum ... and it's a way of also keeping early intervention. It's kind of keeping people out of the mental health services as well, keeping them empowered in their roles, not drifting in to being a patient. (Case manager)

> It would have been nice for me if the job retention team had been involved much earlier on with me. If I had known it was around I would have snatched on it right away because just the little sorts of tips and insights he can give, that would have been much easier. (Employer)

## Client-focused interventions

All 13 clients had received general supportive counselling from their case managers and most commented on how helpful it had been to have someone who was supportive and listened to them, particularly someone outside the situation. Over and above general supportive counselling, the clients had welcomed help in coping with issues such as their working practices, stress or poor attendance. For example:

> I'm a terribly messy worker and if your desk's a mess, you feel a mess. So improving my way of working. (Client)

> So very simple things, like asking for help and admitting that I'm not as strong as I advertise. (Client)

The 13 clients also discussed their job options and preferences with their case manager in terms of whether to return to their current position, consider redeployment within the same organisation or look for new employment. Two clients had no choice as their current employment was terminated and for these two clients, the job retention team intervention involved supporting their claims of unfair dismissal and then supporting them to find new employment.

Four clients chose to leave their current positions and find new employment because they found their work too stressful and their company was unable to offer them redeployment. In these cases the job retention team case manager was reported to be helpful in supporting the clients to reach a decision and explore the types of work that they might consider in the future. The other seven clients chose to return to their workplace. Two were able to negotiate redeployment with the support of their case manager, while five received assistance with negotiating adjustments to their current jobs. These work-focused interventions are considered in more detail later.

Whether clients returned to their original workplace or found a new job, the prospect of returning to work could be daunting and the opportunity to discuss this with their case manager and plan the steps involved was reassuring and helpful.

> The discussions really centred around getting back to work and iden-
> tifying comfort zones and stress zones at work. People I felt happy
> with and the working relationships I had difficulty with. (Client)

In addition to the general support and vocational counselling provided, the majority of clients also received more specific interventions aimed at addressing their particular mental health problems. For example, eight clients reported receiving helpful interventions to improve their management of anxiety. These interventions were quite varied and included meditation, relaxation and alternative therapies. Six clients also described helpful interventions aimed at increasing confidence and assertiveness.

A further key role for the job retention team is to provide ongoing support as necessary for clients who have returned to work. Several clients reported that they found it reassuring to know they could access support should any problems arise once they were back at work, and the support itself was also highly valued.

In four cases the case managers had played a key part in explaining or encouraging the client to explain the mental health problems they were experiencing to family members. As this client explained, their intervention could make a real difference in terms of ensuring family members were supportive.

> My husband thought I should just let the situation go and not
> complain about it and this caused problems between us. It was the
> financial stress. So my case manager briefed him on my state of mind
> and that made a big difference. So then I had support from my
> husband as well. (Client)

Seven clients reported that financial issues were a major concern for them and an added stress contributing to their mental health problems. In these circumstances the case managers' assistance to find ways of coping was also highly valued.

## Work-focused interventions

The work-focused interventions delivered by the job retention team included advocating for the client within the workplace, assistance with legal issues, negotiating adjustments and providing information and support to employers.

Ten clients reported that their case manager had been an advocate for them with their employer, lifting the burden of responsibility for negotiating the resolution of problems. They all reported that this was helpful and many highlighted this aspect of the service as the most helpful intervention they received.

> He took actions when I was unable to. I mean I was saying things
> like, well I'll do this, and he said, that's why I'm here, let me do it for

> you. He's made contact with my line manager and he's also made
> contact, well written, to the head of personnel. He made contact with
> the organisation which I could not do myself. It made the organisa-
> tion sort of come to me and well, I suppose, to meet me in the
> middle. (Client)

Over and above advocacy aimed at resolving problems at work, three clients
reported that their case manager was involved with the legal issues that arose
from their work situations and this support was greatly appreciated whatever
the outcome.

Six clients reported that their case manager had been involved in negotiating
adjustments to facilitate their return to work. The adjustments included moving
into less stressful roles, reducing the hours of work, reducing workloads until
the client's confidence increased and returning to work gradually over a
number of weeks. The clients clearly found this valuable and employers also
reported that it was helpful to have someone suggest and negotiate adjustments
and return to work plans.

> So that disciplinary process reached a head last May where we said
> to the employee after several meetings that we thought the only
> solution was for her to go part-time. She was obviously concerned
> financially but her case manager did a lot of work on her behalf on
> that, and that actually solved the late attendance situation, so it was
> only then just the situation regarding sickness. Her case manager was
> central in helping her relate to our position. (Employer)

As several of the earlier interview extracts indicate, in addition to supporting
their clients, the case managers also provided information and support to help
employers manage employees with mental health problems more effectively.
Although some were wary at first, the five employers who took part in the
research welcomed the job retention team's involvement, for example:

> And the job retention team was there so if I wanted to phone him
> and say I don't know what to do about this, I could. And he would
> suggest to me to think about doing this or maybe think about doing
> that. So I felt some professional support for me as well as for my
> employee. I felt it was more a team, and we were all working
> together working towards a common purpose. I felt that there was a
> support network for me as well. (Employer)

Employers also appreciated an objective perspective on their own concerns
about issues such as the quality or quantity of the employee's work, their level
of sickness absence, extra pressure on other staff members and interpersonal
conflicts in the workplace. In some situations the case manager had a valued
role in mediating and facilitating conversations about these issues between
employee and employer.

> He was an advocate for my employee but he was also very balanced
> and sensible and reasonable. When I met at that meeting, I felt like

at first I handled it very well and then my Irish impatience came and I got upset and so did my employee. He was essential in calming her down and dealing with her. I admire his professionalism and tact. (Employer)

From the case managers' perspective, when employers were willing to engage with the service and participated in supporting a client, the effectiveness of their intervention was all but assured. Across all their clients' employers, however, the job retention team case managers experienced a range of reactions. While some, including those who took part in interviews, were relatively open and supportive, others were more resistant to job retention team intervention, with the result that the case managers had to take a more assertive stance, including highlighting the Disability Discrimination Act and employment law.

I think that probably is the most challenging part when you are in a kind of negative situation with employers, where there has been bullying or harassment or grievance procedures, and it's how much you can kind of get involved in that process and try and regain some control. Often those situations are ones that demand having some knowledge of employment law because if the employers are being discriminating then you have to, there's no other alternative but to tell them what the law says. So they have been some of the most challenging really. (Case manager)

## Outcomes

Seven of the 13 clients who took part in interviews had been able to keep their job with their original organisation. Of these seven clients, three believed they would have lost their job without the job retention team's involvement. The other four clients believed they would have had a more difficult and delayed return to work, which may have resulted in further sickness absence in the future.

I know I wouldn't have returned then. I always felt that if I did not return to work before Christmas then I would be off for a long, long time and I still feel like that now. I couldn't explain to my manager what I needed and I needed a third party to do that talking for me. (Client)

Of the six clients who did not return to their original employer, four had been helped to find another job and two were still looking for work. Five of these six clients thought their mental health would have deteriorated further without the support of the job retention team and three believed their job outcome would have been worse without the job retention team's intervention, either in terms of their financial settlement or their feelings about leaving their company.

Many clients also reported changes in their perspective on work–life balance that they regarded as a positive outcome.

I hate the company that I worked for but they did me a favour. I got out of a place that was no good, blatantly no good, and I have got in to a company with better perks in healthcare, better hours, more money, more holidays, and less responsibilities. I'm more aware of how I react in stressful situations and will take a herbal remedy and sit back and relax. I do manage it better now. I'm contented, I'm happy. I value the friends I have got more now. I value family a whole lot more. Yeah quality time, finding time for myself, finding time for me and the kids and me and the wife. It's an amazing difference. (Client)

Equally, the GPs and employers reported positive outcomes; for example:

My patient found it helpful. This particular person was given advice about the situation at work and what to expect which was great. As well as psychological support and direction that she found valuable. (GP)

I'm not a gambling man but if I was to say, without job retention team involvement she wouldn't be employed now, and I think that 100% you can say that. The employee is certainly a lot more reliable now that she's part-time, which is the major issue as far as we are concerned. There are no unplanned absences. (Employer)

However, one employer did feel that while the service had definitely resulted in the employee retaining his job in the short term, the longer term outcome might still be job termination.

## Conclusion

The AWMHPT job retention service was clearly highly valued by all the people we spoke to and the outcomes achieved during its first year of operation were impressive. All but two of the clients had either returned to their job or found another that suited them better and all 13 clients thought their situation would have been worse had they not been referred to the service. Employers and GPs also highlighted positive outcomes for clients and benefits for themselves.

As Table 14.1 shows, the service met the great majority of the 13 criteria derived from our literature review. Areas where further development might prove useful were providing more general information on healthy workplaces for employers and providing training and advice on employment issues to GPs and mental health workers.

The process of comparing the job retention team with the 13 criteria led to the identification of two additional criteria not identified in the literature and raised questions about one of those that was identified. The two additional criteria concern the inclusion of a focus on relationship issues and family support within the mental health counselling provided and the provision of financial counselling and advice. On the other hand, although a primary allegiance to the client, as recommended in the literature, may be most effective in cases where the employer is not willing to engage with the service, in cases where the employer is willing to engage our results suggest it is important that the case manager remains neutral and offers support to both parties.

**Table 14.1 Comparison with key criteria for an effective job retention service**

| Criterion | AWMHPT Job retention service |
|---|---|
| Vocational counselling – ability to address employment issues, job satisfaction and preference, and disclosure issues without bias and ensuring confidentiality from employer | ✓ |
| Mental health counselling – ability to address mental health issues, symptom management in the workplace, perspectives on illness, psychological detachment from work, and self-esteem and self-identity issues, also ensuring confidentiality | Support on relationship and financial issues may also need to be addressed ✓ |
| Primary allegiance to client | When the employer is willing to engage, a neutral approach may be more effective |
| Advocate for client in the workplace | ✓ |
| Specialist regarding DDA, legal issues and relevant financial incentives or benefits | ✓ |
| Provides training and advice to employers and managers on dealing with mental health issues in the workplace | ✗ |
| Provides training to employers on healthy workplaces for all employees | ✓ |
| Facilitates communication between employee and employer regarding time off work, return to work plans, modified work programmes and adjustments | ✓ |
| Facilitates natural supports within the workplace | ✓ |
| Promotes early intervention and is easily accessible by employers and employees | ✓ |
| Keeps all parties informed – including employer, employee, mental health workers, GPs, etc. | ✓ |
| Ongoing support to manage any problems in the workplace that arise as time goes on | ✓ |
| Provides training and advice on employment issues to mental health workers and GPs | ✗ |

# Chapter 15

# Early intervention: a hand up the slippery slope

Miles Rinaldi and Rachel Perkins

## Introduction

As Tina Thomas and Jenny Secker point out in the previous chapter, early intervention to prevent job loss or enable people to get back to the labour market as quickly as possible is essential if they are not to slide to the bottom of the slippery slope to long-term unemployment and social exclusion. But traditional approaches to helping people with mental health problems gain and retain employment have typically been focused on addressing these needs only after their mental health problems have been addressed through psychopharmacological and psychological interventions. The assumption is that a person has to receive treatment for their symptoms and get better before beginning to look for work. As a result, helping people to return to work begins only, if at all, when a mental health professional has deemed that the person is ready to think about going back to work: for some people this may be after many years.

Traditionally, vocational services have not been integrated into the work of clinical teams and the process of a person engaging with a vocational project has begun when a care coordinator has made a referral to the community vocational resource such as a sheltered work scheme. This is often very late within a person's journey through mental health services. Within that time confidence, self-esteem, self-belief and skills will have diminished and crucially, as Roger Butterworth has shown, a job that the person may have originally held will most likely have been lost.[1]

In essence, mental health services focus on attempting to change the person to fit into society by treating symptoms and developing skills. The notion of recovery – helping people to rebuild a meaningful, satisfying and valued life – is often distant from the reality of services provided. This is far from service users' own priorities. Inspections carried out by the Commission for Health Improvement in 2003 identified that service users' perceptions of the care they needed were often very different from those of the people providing the care.[2] Whereas service users wanted help with employment, housing, social networks, education and a decent income, these were a low priority for services. In 2004 a patient survey carried out by the Healthcare Commission found that 79% of people surveyed were not in paid work and 53% said they had not received any help but would have liked some.[3] The Social Exclusion Unit[4] identified one of the main barriers that people with mental health problems experience when returning to or trying to retain employment as mental health professionals' low expectations of what they could actually achieve. Yet as Patience Seebohm demonstrates in Chapter 8, the role mental health professionals could play in promoting hope and opportunity is crucial if people are going to rebuild a meaningful, satisfying and valued life.

In this chapter we argue that the help service users want to keep or find work needs to be provided at the earliest possible stage in their involvement with services. We begin by looking at the evidence to support that argument and then describe how we are attempting to practise what we preach in South West London.

## Why intervene earlier?

Where health is concerned, studies show that the onset of mental health problems is associated with more than double the risk of leaving employment compared to other health conditions or impairments[5] and becoming unemployed is in turn strongly associated with the development of mental health problems.[6] Once someone has been unemployed for 12 weeks or more, they are at greater risk of depression, anxiety and physical illness than other people.[7] In addition, there is a clear relationship between unemployment and suicide.[8] The risk of suicide is especially high for young men under the age of 35 years, with two-thirds who commit suicide being unemployed.[9] Clinical deterioration among people with a diagnosis of schizophrenia is also significantly associated with lack of occupation.[10]

Yet work itself can improve health. Research shows that employment can lead to improvements in outcome through increasing self-esteem, alleviating psychiatric symptoms and reducing dependency.[11] People with mental health problems who are employed have been found to experience lower levels of symptoms and admission rates to hospital.[12,13] And there are wider benefits for the individual who returns to work. Gary Bond and colleagues found that people with mental health problems in employment showed higher rates of improvement in symptoms, leisure and finances, and self-esteem than people with mental health problems who were unemployed.[14]

The social impact of failing to intervene is also considerable. Unemployment results in decreased social networks and the loss of structure, purpose and identity.[15,16] Contrary to a commonly held belief, Jahoda and her colleagues demonstrated that unemployed people do not exploit the extra time they have available for leisure and social pursuits.[17] Rather, their social networks and social functioning decrease and their motivation and interest reduce, leading to apathy. The Social Exclusion Unit report on mental health and social exclusion[4] confirms the cycle of exclusion that a person with a mental health problem can experience within a short period of time: a single period of hospitalisation or prolonged period of sickness absence from work can lead to unemployment. The report concludes that early intervention is needed to keep people in work.

The evidence regarding the economic impact of failing to intervene is clear: the longer a person is off work, the lower their chance of returning to work. Once someone has been on incapacity benefit for a short period of time we know they have very little chance of returning to work. After six months on incapacity benefit there is a 50% chance of returning to work but this falls to

25% after one year and 10% after two years. Few people return to work after one or two years' absence, irrespective of further treatment.[18]

The costs of a person with mental health problems not working are enormous not only to the individual but also to employers and society. The Sainsbury Centre for Mental Health estimated the total cost of mental health problems to England at £77 billion per year, with output losses associated with missed employment opportunities estimated at over £23 billion per year.[19]

For an individual to be away from the workplace also impacts on their vocational skills and abilities. We live in an age of rapid technological advances within all occupational sectors that directly impacts on the way we work and the types of jobs that are available within the labour market. To disengage from the labour market for lengthy periods of time often results in vocational skills becoming out of date and potentially obsolete. People who are in employment benefit from on-the-job training when new workplace technologies are introduced. They also have the natural support of colleagues who are learning and understanding the new ways of working. However, this opportunity is denied to people who are away from the labour market. Significant periods of absence from the labour market therefore make returning to work that much more difficult.

In addition, the cost to employers is high. Interestingly, when describing the impact of an employee going off sick as a result of mental health problems, employers do not tend to recount stories of people becoming aggressive or behaving in an inappropriate manner at work. Rather, the problems tend to be external to the individual and linked more to the help and support employers themselves receive from health and social services. Employers all too often describe writing to an employee's GP or psychiatrist and finding that it can take several weeks or months to receive a reply. Within that time the employer has incurred significant costs and lost productivity and they are still no wiser as to what is preventing the person from coming back to work. Yet research from the Employers Forum on Disability has shown that retaining a person who develops a mental health problem at work generally costs less than having to recruit and train a new person.[20]

Mental health services can play a key role in reducing the deleterious impact of unemployment by promoting job retention and enabling people who have become unemployed to find work again quickly. To really enable people with mental health problems to succeed in employment, we need to embed employment support into the heart of mental health services, making employment everybody's business. In turn, people with mental health problems would have a much greater chance of remaining in employment because vocational issues would be addressed as part of the overall service they receive and at a time when they really need that support.

## Evidence-based supported employment

Evidence-based supported employment, also known as the Individual, Placement and Support (IPS) approach to vocational rehabilitation for people with severe mental health problems, has been shown to be more effective than other approaches in helping people with mental health problems gain and retain employment (Justine Schneider analyses the research evidence and describes the approach in Chapter 5).

In short, evidence-based supported employment is underpinned by the philosophy that a person is capable of working competitively in the community, if the right kind of job and work environment can be found. Therefore, the primary goal is not to change the individual but to find a natural match between the individual's strengths and experiences and a job in the community, and to provide the support and workplace adjustments they need to make a success of it.

Evidence-based supported employment programmes help anyone who expresses the desire to work. People are not excluded because they are not 'ready' or because of prior work history, substance use or symptoms. Unsurprisingly, people with mental health problems differ from one another in terms of work preferences, the nature of the support they want and the decision whether or not to disclose their mental health problem to the employer or work colleagues. Supported employment programmes respect these individual preferences and tailor their interventions accordingly. This approach means that unlike traditional approaches to vocational rehabilitation, the employment specialist must be integrated into the clinical team. In practice, this means that the individual has access to psychiatrists, psychologists, nurses, social workers and other care providers as well as an employment specialist. Therefore all staff within the clinical team collaborate to provide optimal support.

## Evidence in practice

At South West London and St George's Mental Health NHS Trust, vocational services and occupational therapy staff have developed vocational services within the community mental health teams (CMHTs) designed to provide the assistance that clients need to access and retain work and education. Insofar as resources allow, the model adopted is based on the research evidence. In particular, vocational support is integrated into the work of the clinical teams, there is a focus on enabling people to access work and education in open, integrated, settings, people are provided with support as part of their care plans to maintain their work/study and there is a focus on individual user preferences. The role of occupational therapy has been important in the delivery of the services.[21]

The approach comprises three elements.

1. Occupational therapists are the designated clinical vocational leads within teams and have at least one session per week dedicated to fulfilling this role, both in direct work with clients and in providing advice and support to other team members in relation to vocational issues.
2. The occupational therapy leads work in conjunction with trained employment specialists whose role is to provide a specialist vocational resource to staff and clients within the team. In April 2003 there were 4.5 employment specialists in post working with CMHTs. By March 2004 this had increased to nine. The employment specialists have the specific remit of linking with local employers, the JobCentre Plus and Disability Employment advisors, mainstream employment and training services, specialist employment and

training services for people with mental health problems run by other agencies, colleges and other education providers; assisting in vocational assessments; helping clients to access the opportunities that are available; and assisting care coordinators in providing ongoing support. The evidence base would indicate that there is a need for one employment specialist per CMHT but it has not yet been possible to achieve this in all areas.
3. Individual care coordinators provide ongoing support in work/education for clients, with assistance from the team employment specialists and occupational therapy staff as necessary.

In addition, employment specialists and occupational therapy staff work closely with the trust's Welfare Rights Service to provide welfare benefits advice to those wishing to enter work and education.

And it works. In the year April 2003 to March 2004 the approach achieved impressive results.[22]*

- One thousand, one hundred and eighty-two people received specific vocational input whose primary goal was to assist them to obtain work (open employment or mainstream voluntary work) or education/training in mainstream integrated settings.
- The majority of these people had more serious and complex mental health problems: 97% were on enhanced level care planning; 60% had a diagnosis of some form of psychosis; and 67% had been in contact with the CMHT for more than one year.
- Prior to intervention, only 261 of these people (22%) were engaged in work/study in a mainstream integrated setting and 687 people (58%) were completely unoccupied.
- During 2003–4, 650 people (55%) were supported to gain or maintain work/study in a mainstream integrated setting:
  - the number of people engaged in open employment rose from 125 (11%) to 271(23%)
  - the number engaged in mainstream education/training increased from 88 (7%) to 222 (19%)
  - the number engaged in mainstream voluntary work rose from 48 (4%) to 157 (13%).

Since people with mental health problems are at double the risk of losing their jobs as a consequence of their mental health problems, helping people to retain work was very important. Of the 125 people who were in employment at the start of the intervention, 104 were assisted to retain their employment, a retention rate of 83%.

Whilst the results of the interventions are impressive, it should be noted that just under two-thirds of those people who received a specific intervention had been in contact with the clinical teams for one year or more. Even so, people were receiving a specific vocational intervention much faster than they traditionally would have done.

* Results are for the calendar year; individuals had received a service for between one and 29 months.

It is often assumed that employment, mainstream education/training and mainstream voluntary work/work experience are only suitable for those with less serious mental health problems. However, the vocational outcomes achieved here run counter to this belief.

- There was no significant association between length of contact with the CMHT and either vocational status at the start of the intervention or whether the person was successful in engaging in work/study in an open, integrated setting as a result of the intervention.
- There was no significant association between the severity/complexity of a person's needs – as indicated by whether they were on enhanced or standard level care planning (CPA) – and either vocational status at the start of the intervention or whether the person was successful in engaging in work/study in an open, integrated setting as a result of the intervention.
- There was a significant association between diagnosis and vocational status at the start of the intervention. Those with a diagnosis of some form of psychosis were significantly less likely to be engaged in work/study in a mainstream integrated setting at the start than those with a non-psychotic diagnosis (19.5% compared with 25%).
- However, diagnosis did not have an impact on the outcomes of intervention. The proportion of people with a psychotic diagnosis engaged in work/study in a mainstream integrated setting following intervention (53.8%) did not differ significantly from the proportion of people with a non-psychotic diagnosis (56.6%).
- The proportion of people with a psychotic diagnosis who were engaged in:
  - open employment increased from 8.6% to 22.2%
  - mainstream education/training increased from 6.8% to 18.2%
  - mainstream voluntary work/work experience increased from 3.9% to 13.3%.
- The proportion of people with a non-psychotic diagnosis engaged in:
  - open employment increased from 14.3% to 24.1%
  - mainstream education/training increased from 7.8% to 19.4%
  - mainstream voluntary work/work experience increased from 4.2% to 13.1%.

These findings confirm the results of previous research. In his review of the research evidence, Gary Bond clearly shows that supported employment studies have failed to find any relationship between diagnosis, symptomatology and disability status and employment outcomes.[23]

# Early intervention for young people with first-episode psychosis

An example of an even earlier vocational intervention can be found in the work of the trust's Early Intervention in Psychosis Service. Early intervention services provide community-based treatment and support to young people with psychosis and their families, with an emphasis on maintaining normal social roles.[24] Birchwood and colleagues identified a vocational outcome as a central aim of the recovery process for such services.[25] Employment rates for this group tend to follow a similar pattern and when they first come into contact with services a proportion will be in competitive employment. However, within one year employment rates tend to drop dramatically, in one study from 52% to 25%.[26] The centrality of an early vocational intervention to these services is clear.

In South West London, a half-time vocational specialist was integrated into the early intervention team to provide evidence-based supported employment, thus addressing the vocational needs of clients within the service. As the average age of these people was 21 years, education is as important as employment. Within six months of the intervention the proportion of clients in employment rose from 10% to 28% and by 12 months to 40%. The proportion in education remained constant at 33% for the first six months, with clients then moving into competitive employment. Only one client remained without any form of vocational activity. It is important to note that the vocational specialist was not only assisting people to gain employment and education but also addressing the issue of job or course retention. Seventeen clients (43%) were engaged in employment or education at the time of their referral to the service and the vocational specialist along with the team supported all of these clients to retain this.[27]

## Benefits of integrated clinical and vocational services

As Justine Schneider's analysis of the research evidence in Chapter 5 shows, integrated clinical and vocational services achieve better employment outcomes. Integrated services offer four consistent advantages over non-integrated services.[28]

- More effective vocational and clinical engagement and retention.
- Better communication between vocational staff and clinical staff to the benefit of the individual who is retaining or returning to work.
- Opportunities for clinicians to understand and focus on employment.
- Incorporation of clinical information into vocational plans and services.

An overarching benefit is that clinicians, rather than the individual themselves, take responsibility for the coordination, consistency and coherence of the vocational service received.

## Conclusion

As we saw at the beginning of this chapter, the Social Exclusion Unit report on social exclusion and mental health identified the low expectations of health and social care staff about what people with mental health problems can achieve as a major barrier to inclusion.[4] If people are to be able to take control of their lives and build a future for themselves, hope and opportunity are essential. Without hope – if you are unable to see the possibility of a decent future for yourself – then it is not possible to set about the task of rebuilding your life. But without

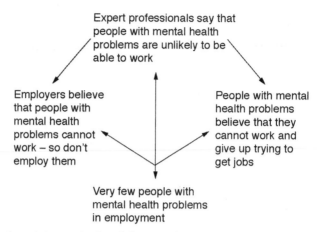

Figure 15.1: The vicious circle of despondency.

opportunity – if everywhere you turn you are denied access to the things that you value, the things that give your life meaning – you are prevented from rebuilding a meaningful and valued life.

The problem is that the low expectations of mental health professionals set up a vicious circle that erodes hope and diminishes opportunity and that is then reinforced throughout society. For example, if mental health professionals, regarded within society as experts, say that people with mental health problems are unlikely to be able to work then this has two effects:

- people with mental health problems believe them and give up trying to get jobs: 'If the experts say I cannot work then what hope is there?'
- employers believe them and are reluctant to employ people: 'If the experts say they cannot work, then what is the point in employing them?'.

If people with mental health problems give up applying for jobs and employers stop employing them then this guarantees that there will be very few people with mental health problems in employment. Then everyone can say 'I told you so' in a vicious circle of despondency. In this situation, as Figure 15.1 illustrates, it is really no wonder that there are so few people with mental health problems in employment.

If services are to promote independence, enabling people to do the things they want to do and make the most of their skills, then the vicious circle of despondency must be replaced by a virtuous circle of optimism.

Irrespective of the theories we hold about the nature and origins of mental distress and disability, we need to move away from prescribing what is good for people towards enabling people to take control of their own lives. In relation to employment, the challenge remains to move from opinion-based practice to intervening earlier through evidence-based practice. Our experience in South West London shows it can be done.

# References

1 Butterworth R (2001) Job retention – developing a service. *Mental Health Review.* **6**(4): 17–20.

2 Commission for Health Improvement (2003) *What CHI has found in Mental Health Trusts.* Commission for Health Improvement, London.

3 Healthcare Commission (2004) *Patient Survey Report 2004, Mental Health.* Healthcare Commission, London.

4 ODPM (2004) *Mental Health and Social Exclusion.* Social Exclusion Unit Report. Office of the Deputy Prime Minister, London.

5 Burchardt T (2003) *Employment Retention and the Onset of Sickness or Disability: evidence from the Labour Force Survey longitudinal datasets.* Department for Work and Pensions, report no.109, London.

6 Warr P (1987) *Unemployment and Mental Health.* Oxford University Press, Oxford.

7 Department for Work and Pensions (2003) *Pathways to Work: helping people into employment.* The Stationery Office, Norwich.

8 Lewis G and Sloggett A (1998) Suicide, deprivation and unemployment: record linkage study. *British Medical Journal.* **317**: 1283–6.

9 Department of Health (2001) *Safety First: five year report of the national confidential inquiry into suicide and homicide by people with mental illness.* Department of Health, London.

10 Wing J and Brown G (1970) *Institutionalism and Schizophrenia: a comparative study of three mental hospitals.* Cambridge University Press, London.

11 Cook J and Razzano L (2000) Vocational rehabilitation for persons with schizophrenia: recent research and implications for practice. *Schizophrenia Bulletin.* **26**(1): 87–103.

12 Brown G, Carstairs G and Topping G (1958) Post-hospital adjustment of chronic mental patients. *Lancet.* **2**: 685–9.

13 Warner R (1994) *Recovery from Schizophrenia, Psychiatry and Political Economy* (2e). Routledge and Kegan Paul, London.

14 Bond G, Resnick S, Drake R *et al.* (2001) Does competitive employment improve non-vocational outcomes for people with severe mental illness? *Journal of Consulting and Clinical Psychology.* **69**(3): 489–501.

15 Bennett D (1970) The value of work in psychiatric rehabilitation. *Social Psychiatry.* **5**: 224–30.

16 Collis M and Ekdawi M (1984) Social adjustments in rehabilitation. *International Journal of Rehabilitation Research.* **7**: 259–72.

17 Jahoda M, Lazarsfeld P and Zeisl H (1933) *Marienthal: the sociography of an unemployed community.* Tavistock Publications, London.

18 Clinical Standards Advisory Group (1994) *Back Pain.* HMSO, London.

19 Sainsbury Centre for Mental Health (2003) *Economic and Social Costs of Mental Illness in England.* Sainsbury Centre for Mental Health, London.

20 Scott-Parker S and Zadek S (2001) *Unlocking the Evidence: the new disability business case.* Employers Forum on Disability, London.

21 Davis M and Rinaldi M (2004) Using an evidence-based approach to enable people with mental health problems to gain and retain employment, education and voluntary work. *British Journal of Occupational Therapy.* **67**: 319–22.

22 Rinaldi M, Morris J and Perkins R (2004) *Adult Services: vocational services in community mental health teams, annual report, April 2003–March 2004.* South West London and St George's Mental Health NHS Trust, London.

23 Bond G (2004) Supported employment: evidence for an evidence-based practice. *Psychiatric Rehabilitation Journal.* **27**: 345–59.

24 Department of Health (2001) *The Mental Health Policy Implementation Guide.* Department of Health, London.

25 Birchwood M, McGorry P and Jackson H (1997) Early intervention in schizophrenia. *British Journal of Psychiatry.* **170**(1): 2–11.

26 Birchwood M, Cochrane R, Macmillan F *et al.* (1992) The influence of ethnicity and family structure on relapse in first episode schizophrenia: a comparison of Asian, Afro-Caribbean and White patients. *British Journal of Psychiatry.* **161**: 783–90.

27 Rinaldi M, McNeil K, Firn M *et al.* (2004) What are the benefits of evidence-based supported employment for patients with first episode psychosis? *Psychiatric Bulletin.* **28**(8): 281–4.

28 Bond G, Drake R, Mueser K *et al.* (1997) An update on supported employment for people with mental illness. *Psychiatric Services.* **48**: 335–46.

# Conclusion: the end of all our exploring ...

Bob Grove, Jenny Secker and Patience Seebohm

The preceding chapters have presented a wealth of evidence that we hope will inform and inspire a paradigm shift within mental health services: a shift from a narrow, medical view of mental distress to a perspective that recognises strengths and abilities as well as needs, that inspires hope and encourages the fulfilment of people's potential.

The evidence from the research we and other contributors have reviewed and carried out leaves no room for doubt that the majority of people who need to use mental health services want to work, and that wanting to work is the only qualification required for them to succeed, given the right job and appropriate support. There is much evidence, too, about what that support entails. For those wanting to return to the labour market after a period of unemployment: a focus on real, paid jobs; attention to people's own ambitions; finding a job that matches those ambitions as well as meeting other needs; and support in work for as long as is necessary. For those in employment at the point of first contact with services: early intervention to prevent job loss; case management aimed at designing and implementing a back-to-work plan, with the involvement of the employer where possible; and, again, support in work for as long as it is needed.

When faced with the need for a fundamental shift in thinking, a natural response is to throw up a screen of criticism in the hope of deflecting the wave of change – we have all done it. One such criticism of the research evidence is that so many of the key studies were carried out in the United States, giving us the excuse that we don't know whether it will work in the UK and meanwhile, should we not play safe? While further research here is certainly required, ground-breaking service development is already demonstrating that employment support and job retention services can and do work in the UK. The contributions of Rachel Perkins, Miles Rinaldi and Tina Thomas demonstrate that clearly.

More powerfully still, the chapters contributed by others with experience of using mental health services both reinforce and add to the international research evidence. We learn at first hand from these authors how important work is in making us feel valued (and therefore valuable), in providing social contact and, in Mo Hutchison's words, simply 'keeping us going'. We also learn how the wrong job can contribute to or compound mental health problems when managers and colleagues are unsupportive and feedback isn't given about how we are doing. Although evidence-based employment support is not yet widely available in the UK, some contributors have been fortunate to receive, and to give others, support that closely approximates to it. For Paul Grey and

John Marshall, a focus on enabling people to articulate and achieve their own goals is paramount, as is the confidence building and support in work described by Jo Shenton and Richard Watts.

We also learn from these chapters some lessons not encompassed within the research literature that reinforce the need for a paradigm shift. A strong theme in many chapters is the centrality of family support. Historically in the UK, family members have been regarded with some suspicion by mental health professionals as part of the problem or even the cause of the problem. More recently, they have been designated 'carers', to be recruited as allies and assessed for support in their own right.[1] Obviously that is an advance but still the rhetoric smacks of a division between 'user' and 'carer', both now corralled in narrow, professionally designated roles. As Paul Grey illustrates, we need to understand people in their family context and recognise that family members may be confused and concerned about changes they do not understand because they have been offered no information. Interestingly, Paul's point also emerged from the evaluation of the Avon and Wiltshire job retention service described in Chapter 14. As we move forward in developing employment services in the UK, it is a point we must keep to the forefront of our minds.

But not everyone has close family, or family close enough, to offer support in achieving their ambitions and in any case, we all need friends outside the family circle. In their own ways, Graham Cockshutt, Paul Grey, Mo Hutchison and Mary Nettle all graphically illustrate how service users themselves can support each other, through self-help groups established for mutual support or as role models and mentors showing each other what can be achieved and helping each other achieve it. Far from being the passive recipients of our evidence-based services, service users have a wealth of knowledge and experience to offer each other. Our task as professionals is to ensure this expertise is put at the centre of our services. Our role as professionals is to be, as Graham Cockshutt puts it, 'supporting actors'.

Thinking differently about the jobs people might do is a further challenge highlighted by these authors, many of whom are running their own businesses. So often, as Paul Grey himself has found, we think only of entry-level jobs when considering people's potential. Inevitably, we also share with Richard Watts the notions of a 'proper job' that are so firmly embedded in our culture. Like Richard, though, we need to break out of those cultural constraints and recognise that while entry-level jobs may be ideal for some people, self-employment may offer others the fertile ground they need to flourish.

We were tempted to give this final chapter a title that would summarise the shift in thinking and practice we believe is necessary if people who use mental health services are to lead the kind of lives they want and are entitled to expect as citizens of our nation. We thought of 'From Here to Equality', because implicit in our exploration of the links between mental distress, employment and social exclusion has been the necessity of shifting the balance of power from service providers to service users. However, someone got there first and not wanting to be confused with the National Institute for Mental Health England,[2] we ruled it out. We also thought of 'Give Them The Money', a title borrowed from a (slightly) tongue-in-cheek article by Bob Grove[3] in which he suggested that if all the money spent on day services were simply given to service users, then they would probably make a pretty good fist of leading decent lives without the need for professionalised care. However, even this is not exactly a new idea and one could argue that direct payments are already heading in that direction.[4] This is the trouble with new thinking – it almost always turns out not to be new at all.

In the end, we settled for borrowing from the poet T S Eliot:[5]

> We shall not cease from exploration
> And the end of all our exploring
> Will be to arrive where we started
> And know the place for the first time.

We hope that some or even most of what the contributors to this book have said rings bells, sounds familiar, has been 'lost and found and lost again and again'.[6] What then is it that prevents us dealing with the wasteful and unnecessary journey towards disempowerment, unemployment and social exclusion that is the experience of so many people who use mental health services? The answer lies in the insidious power of institutional thinking. Because we have closed the large mental institutions, it does not follow that we have got rid of the institutionalising processes that go on in our heads. For this, we need an alternative way of looking at the world – and a daemon with sharp critical faculties that sits on our shoulders and nags at us when we slip into sloppy, empty slogans that give new ideas the properties of the status quo.

Take the shift in the balance of power between professionals and service users, for instance. We talk of participation and consultation but rarely of commissioning and control – particularly of the finances. Very few professionals indeed have got to the point of accepting the role of 'supporting actor' and yet the case for such a shift is very persuasive when viewed from the perspective of the recovering survivor. Using the new paradigm helps us move beyond these artificial barriers, described by Paul Grey as 'the old governing principles', and not only in theory. One of us was privileged to play a small role in a daring example of shifting power relations, described by Rob Hughes as the 'Aberdeen 50/50 approach to service development and commissioning'.[7] This, in essence, was a successful attempt to get beyond tokenism and share with the service users themselves the responsibility for transforming an out-of-date (and very expensive) industrial therapy unit into a comprehensive local employment service. One of the lessons for the service users was that true partnership brings with it responsibilities and tough decisions. Rob concludes by saying:

> I am not sure if we have opened Pandora's Box or let the genie out of the bottle but either way there is no going back. Thankfully the 50/50 approach is becoming increasingly accepted as the goal for all future service user involvement in the development of new services.

We hope that if you have got this far, you will share our belief that the new paradigm in which professionals collaborate with service users to undertake the journey to recovery and active citizenship is not Pandora's Box but the beginning of an exciting exploration of the possible.

What then are the practical implications – the must dos – if we are to achieve the necessary shift in the way services are organised? What follows is a series of precepts and ideas that seem to us a distillation of the essential points of the new paradigm and its application.

- First, we should rule no one out of programmes to aid employment and recovery. Trying to sort out the employable sheep from the unemployable goats is wasted effort. Far better to concentrate on giving everyone the kind of help they, as individuals, want and need.
- People are not mad all the time, so they and we who support them should concentrate much more on who they are and what they can do when they are well. Illness is only a part of life and not the most important part. As for anyone else, a valued role, family and friends are the important things.
- People gain in courage and strength from association with others who have had similar experiences. Professionals must learn the skill of knowing when to take a back seat and becoming 'supporting actors' even where the demands of a risk-averse system make this difficult. There should be more experimentation with direct payments, funded self-help groups, community development approaches and so on that shift the balance of power and look for solutions in people's own lives and collective experience. As John Marshall reminds us in Chapter 12, 'A ship is safe in harbour but that is not what it is made for'.
- This does not mean ignoring or skimping on mental health services. People will only be able to undertake the recovery journey if they know they can rely on their psychiatrist or CPN or social worker to intervene where necessary in a timely fashion and to offer practical and emotional support for their ambitions when they are well.
- Mental health professionals have a profound influence on people's self-confidence and on what others think they are capable of. It is therefore a duty to be positive and to find ways of offering hope to patients, relatives and employers even where the apparent prognosis is not good. This is not only a duty but a skill and it is a skill that should be at the core of all professional training curricula.
- Research programmes using the new paradigm as a conceptual base should be funded by the government, the research councils and the large grant-making foundations. Perhaps a levy for such research from the pharmaceutical industry on the profits from high-selling psychotropic medication would be a way of redressing the present imbalance between drug trials and studies of psychosocial interventions.
- And finally we will all need to keep going – challenging, experimenting, learning the lessons of failure as well as success, finding out what is possible. As Rachel Perkins (with the help of Geoff Shepherd's 'turning a tanker' simile) has demonstrated in Chapter 9, there is an entire system out there and it will not be changed overnight. It *can* be changed, however, and it can be changed by lots of people taking small steps, working in different ways, spreading new possibilities within their own professional groups, finding a new settlement between risk and safety.

As you will have spotted, the title of the concluding chapter is not an end at all, it is just a beginning.

# References

1 Department of Health (2002) *Developing Services for Carers and Families of People with Mental Illness.* Department of Health, London.

2 National Institute for Mental Health England (2004) *From Here to Equality.* National Institute for Mental Health England, Leeds.

3 Grove B (1998) Give them the money – a modest proposal for abolishing day care. *Mental Health Practice.* 2(1): 9–11.

4 Information about this means of purchasing services can be found at www.direct.gov.uk.

5 Eliot T S (2001) *Four Quartets. Number 4: Little Gidding.* Faber and Faber, London.

6 Eliot T S (2001) *Four Quartets. Number 2: East Coker.* Faber and Faber, London.

7 Hughes R (2000) The Aberdeen 50/50 approach to service development and commissioning. *A Life in the Day.* 4(4): 12–15.

# Chapter 2

# What do service users want?

Patience Seebohm and Jenny Secker

## Introduction

As Bob Grove and Helen Membrey pointed out in the previous chapter, there is a deeply embedded assumption within mental health services that service users do not want to work. In 1996 Peter Bates published a ground-breaking study that challenged that assumption.[1] Of 77 day centre clients interviewed for the study, 47 (61%) said they wanted help to return to work, and this despite having been in contact with mental health services for an average of 21 years. A few years later, Miles Rinaldi and Robert Hill published similar results from a survey of disabled people, including people with mental health problems, in Merton, South West London.[2] Of 127 people who were not currently working, almost half of whom had a mental health problem, 63 (51%), wanted to return to work, including 23 people who reported having been advised not to work by a health professional. In total, 55 people had been given similar advice.

In order to build on these studies, we wanted to focus more specifically on people with mental health problems than was possible in the Merton study and to include a broader range of people than those using day centres. In 1999 a grant from the English Department of Health combined with funds from the local mental health NHS trust provided the opportunity to do so in the city of Sheffield. The aim was to identify service users' employment, training and education goals, the barriers they faced in achieving them and the help they felt they needed to overcome these. Through doing so, we also hoped to raise the profile of vocational needs among mental health professionals.

To practise what we were preaching, we recruited eight people with experience of using mental health services as interviewers. Regular support, training and supervision were provided on visits to Sheffield and over the telephone. The interviewers were paid an hourly rate above the minimum wage plus expenses. To ensure benefits regulations were not infringed, payment was made in ways to suit individual circumstances.

One hundred and fifty-six service users took part in the survey. Although the survey questions were answered by ticking the appropriate box or boxes, the interviews were conversational in style and participants were invited to add comments, which were noted on the questionnaire. Following completion of the survey, it was clear that certain groups of people were underrepresented, particularly people of African and African Caribbean heritage, Asian women and men in the 50–65 age group. Focus group discussions were therefore convened to explore the issues raised in the survey with these groups. The groups considered two issues: the difficulties experienced in taking up education, training or work; and the solutions required to overcome those difficulties.

In this chapter we first describe what the survey participants were currently doing during the day, their aspirations for the future and the kind of help they had received or wanted to achieve then. Drawing on both the survey and focus group data, we then look at the barriers participants faced and the solutions they proposed to overcome them. Because the survey questions allowed people to select more than one answer to reflect the multiplicity of their current activities and aspirations, the percentages in our tables add up to more than 100%.

## Current daytime activities

Table 2.1 shows the current daytime activities reported by interview participants. Of the seven service users in open employment, four were in full-time jobs and three in part-time jobs. Nearly a quarter of participants were not engaged in any regular activity.

Table 2.1  Daytime activities

| Activity | % (n) |
| --- | --- |
| Day centre | 44.9 (70) |
| Drop-in | 28.2 (44) |
| Education/training | 17.9 (28) |
| Sheltered work | 14.1 (22) |
| Voluntary work | 12.8 (20) |
| Open employment | 4.5 (7) |
| Work experience in an open setting | 1.3 (2) |
| No regular activity | 23.1 (36) |

## Future aspirations

The 149 service users who were not already in paid employment were asked if they were interested in obtaining work of any kind, including voluntary work. They had the opportunity to respond positively (yes), more tentatively (maybe in the future) or negatively (no). Only 15 people (10%) had no interest in any kind of work. Their reasons revolved largely around their illness itself, their medication, discrimination or concerns about coming off or jeopardising welfare benefits. When asked if they would like to take up some kind of education or training, eight of the 15 people also had no interest in either, while five expressed definite interest in this option. Two people expressed more tentative interest.

Participants who expressed an interest in work, education or training, whether positive or tentative ($n = 141$), were asked to select the opportunities they would like from a given list. Since none of the opportunities are mutually exclusive, they could select as many opportunities as they wished. As Table 2.2 illustrates, the great majority of people, almost 97%, identified paid work, whether full-time, part-time or self-employed, as a clear aspiration, in addition to or in preference to other goals.

Table 2.2 Preferred opportunities

| Vocational opportunity | % (n) |
|---|---|
| Paid employment (full-time, part-time or self-employed | 95.7 (132) |
| Education or training | 68.8 (97) |
| Voluntary work | 61.6 (85) |
| Work experience (in open job market) | 48.6 (67) |
| Supported work | 44.2 (61) |
| Job preparation courses | 26.2 (37) |
| Other | 16.7 (23) |
| Don't know | 2.1 (3) |

## Help received and wanted

Participants with an interest in work, education or training were also asked whether they had received any vocational assistance. Seventy-five people (53%) had not received any help. Those who had received help were asked to identify the source(s) from a given list. Table 2.3 shows the sources of assistance they identified. A third of the participants had received help from sources other than those on the list. These included college, family and friends.

Table 2.3 Sources of assistance

| Source | % (n) |
|---|---|
| Community psychiatric nurse | 30.3 (20) |
| Day centre and/or development officer | 22.7 (15) |
| Employment advisor (DEA/job centre) | 19.7 (13) |
| Social worker | 16.7 (11) |
| Voluntary organisation | 13.6 (9) |
| Occupational therapist | 12.1 (8) |
| Careers office | 9.1 (6) |
| Nurse (not CPN) | 3.0 (2) |
| Other | 34.8 (23) |

Whether or not they had previously received vocational assistance, participants were asked whether they would like such help in the future. Twenty-five service users (18%) wanted no assistance but 116 (82%) either definitely (62%) or tentatively (20%) wanted help. Those already in education and training were particularly anxious to obtain help, with 14 of the 18 people concerned identifying this as a need.

The 116 service users who wanted assistance were asked about the kind of help they wanted. Again, they could choose as many options as they wished from a given list. As Table 2.4 shows, continuing or improved help with mental health problems was most important to them.

**Table 2.4 Preferred vocational assistance**

| Type of assistance | % (n) |
|---|---|
| Help for mental health/keep current service | 71.5 (83) |
| Advice on how benefits will be affected | 61.2 (71) |
| Help for mental health/get better services | 50.9 (59) |
| Support to keep paid employment | 49.1 (57) |
| Advice and help to get training | 45.6 (54) |
| Work experience (in ordinary job setting) | 45.7 (53) |
| Help to find and stay in education | 43.1 (50)) |
| Help to find paid employment | 41.4 (48) |
| Training on preparing for a job | 40.5 (47) |
| Careers advice and counselling | 37.9 (44) |
| Help and advice on self-employment | 15.5 (18) |
| Help with caring for others | 8.6 (10) |
| Don't know | 5.2  (6) |

## Barriers and solutions

All 156 service users who took part in the survey were asked to select the most significant barriers to the employment of people with mental health problems from a given list. Participants could select as many options as they wished. Table 2.5 summarises their responses.

**Table 2.5 Barriers to employment**

| Barrier | % (n) |
|---|---|
| Employer attitudes | 83 (129) |
| Mental health problems | 80 (124) |
| Benefits system | 69 (107) |
| Lack of work experience | 54  (84) |
| Lack of support | 53  (83) |
| Lack of skills or qualifications | 51  (79) |
| Age | 50  (78) |
| Lack of vacancies | 49  (77) |
| Public transport (availability or difficulty using) | 30  (47) |
| Caring for others | 17  (27) |
| Other | 15  (23) |

As the table illustrates, discrimination on the part of employers, mental health problems and inflexibility within the welfare benefits system were perceived to be the main barriers and these results were echoed in the focus group discussions. Everyone who took part in the groups perceived the fear of losing benefits coupled with a lack of impartial advice as a major barrier to employment, education or training. People from the African and African Caribbean communities were particularly concerned that leaving benefits for a paid job would not be worthwhile for people living in supported housing, where rents were high as a result of the additional support costs, and men in the 50–65-age group were also concerned about the difficulty of earning a wage higher than benefit levels. This group also highlighted the potential difficulty of returning to benefits if necessary.

Many focus group participants also described the stigma attached to mental ill health and the resulting discrimination as a major barrier. Experiences of stigmatisation, which sapped their confidence and motivation to move on in terms of vocational activities, were reported to be a constant feature of their lives. For the African and African Caribbean participants, both institutional and personal racism greatly compounded this problem. Equally, some of the Asian women reported experiencing ignorance and stigma about mental ill health at college while attending English as a Second Language courses and for most of the women in this group, inadequate language teaching was an additional barrier. The older men's group also felt employers would discriminate on the basis of both their age and health problems.

In terms of solutions, reliable advice and information were a high priority for all the groups that took part in the research. Needs here included:

- impartial, trustworthy advice about benefits from people who understand both the benefits system and mental health and employment issues
- expert careers advice, again from people with an understanding of mental health and employment issues
- information about opportunities provided in day centres through talks and written material
- the provision of information in community languages.

Where tackling stigma and discrimination was concerned, the older men's group thought responsibility lay with the government to strengthen the Disability Discrimination Act and to ensure that public services did not discriminate against people with mental health problems. The creation of employment opportunities was a high priority for most people and for many, this meant starting 'at home', in the NHS and local authority services. However, the creation of opportunities alone was not seen as sufficient. In addition, professional employment support from people knowledgeable about both mental health and employment issues was regarded as essential. Although some groups valued opportunities for job preparation, including voluntary work, the emphasis was on the need for 'real work'. For the older men and participants from the African and African Caribbean communities in particular, sheltered work which appeared to offer 'real work' but without competitive wages was not considered an acceptable option.

The creation of opportunities for education and training, again with ongoing professional support, was also seen as important and was highlighted as a priority by the African and African Caribbean participants. Among participants in the older men's group too, education appealed to many, once it was understood this could be very different from earlier experiences. The men identified interests they would like to pursue through some kind of study, such as local history and architecture. They also felt they would benefit from learning practical living skills such as cooking. For the Asian women's group, the provision of adequate, appropriate childcare was clearly a prerequisite to taking up employment and educational opportunities.

## Conclusion

Only half the survey participants were involved in any vocational activity, with only seven people in paid work, yet a huge majority, almost 96%, wanted to obtain paid employment at some point in the future. It is not possible to be certain why this is so much higher than the 51–61% reported in previous surveys but it is likely that asking participants about more tentative as well as current aspirations may have encouraged people with lower levels of confidence to express their hopes and dreams.

Participants in both the survey and the focus groups called for a range of positive, practical measures to help them on their way to achieving their goals. Survey participants highlighted gaining skills through work experience of different types as important, together with specialist mental health employment support and guidance. However, over half had received no help at all from any source, and occupational therapists, who might be expected to have a specialist vocational role, did not feature as a source of advice or support for the great majority of people. Yet participants looked to mental health services to challenge the barriers they faced. The great majority identified continuing mental health support as the most important requirement for people wanting to move on in terms of vocational activity, suggesting that mental health services should fit around their working lives rather than delivering support only to those who are unemployed. Many participants in both the survey and focus groups spoke of the need for mental health services to make links with the employment world, directly helping service users into paid jobs, and to set an example themselves by ensuring employment opportunities are available to service users. In this context, addressing discrimination was seen as key, including the multiple discrimination in the workplace faced by people from black and minority ethnic groups and by older people.

Since the survey was carried out, some progress has been made in addressing many of the barriers identified by the service users we spoke to. At the national level, flexibilities have been introduced to welfare benefit regulations that enable people who come off incapacity benefits to reclaim the benefit, if the need arises, within one year. In addition, new Permitted Work rules clarify the situation of people who do part-time paid work as a way of gaining work experience. As well as being able to earn the national minimum wage for up to 16 hours per week, the new rules treat them as proper employees with all the rights that pertain. However, as with the previous Therapeutic Earnings, those on means-tested benefits can work for only four hours a week on a paid basis before they start to lose benefits. Our experience is that many service users are unaware of these changes and those who do know about them find them very difficult to understand, highlighting a continuing need for expert, impartial advice that is still not widely available. Service users who return to work still face risk to their income and a dilemma between working a very small number of hours each week or increasing their hours substantially to maintain their income, potentially at the expense of their mental health. The Disability Alliance has published a guide specifically to help mental health professionals improve the advice they give to service users thinking of returning to work.[3]

Also at the national level, in 2002 the Department of Health published guidance aimed at increasing the employment of people with mental health problems within the NHS[4] while a 2002 amendment to the Disability Discrimination Act of 1995 extends the Act's provisions to educational institutions. If enacted, a further amendment published in 2003 will place a duty to promote disability equality on the public sector, and proposals to address age discrimination at work were also published in 2003. At present, however, initiatives aimed at increasing employment with appropriate support within the NHS are rare, the exemplar project in South West London being a notable exception (*see* Chapters 9 and 15). In addition, the draft Disability Discrimination Bill of 2003 does not address concerns about the 1995 Act, which requires that people with mental health problems, unlike any other disability group, must have 'a clinically well-recognised illness' that is long term and has 'a substantial adverse effect on normal day-to-day activities'. As the national mental health organisation, Mind, points out,[5] these requirements create inequality between people with mental health problems and other groups, and exclude problems which may not be continuous and long term but rather recede and recur over time. Moreover, the assessment of impact on day-to-day activities is based on a list of activities that is largely irrelevant to mental health. And, of course, in order to exercise their rights, people must be aware of them, but many mental health service users remain unaware that disability discrimination legislation applies to them[6] (*see* Chapter 13 for more on this).

At the local level, as Justine Schneider shows in Chapter 6, access to combined mental health and employment support remains limited for mental health service users. However, this is now a greater priority following publication of the Social Exclusion Unit's report on mental health and social exclusion.[7] In this context, the involvement of occupational therapists is likely to increase from the relatively low levels identified in Sheffield, and in that city has already done so. As Miles Rinaldi and Rachel Perkins point out in their contributions to this book, that has certainly been the case in South West London, where the occupational therapist's role has proved particularly valuable.

In employing service users as interviewers, our research project itself provides evidence of the valuable resource represented by people who use mental health services. All the interviewers proved to be committed and skilled and the study benefited greatly from their involvement, as research in the US suggests.[8] The recruitment of service users attracted support and interest from interviewees and staff, ensuring that employment issues were highlighted in a positive way. Partly due to the impact of this survey, a user employment project is now well established at the NHS mental health trust in Sheffield and one of the service user researchers has obtained paid work running the project in partnership with an occupational therapist.

Thus the survey has demonstrated how unthinking assumptions about service users have led mental health services to ignore the importance of employment aspirations in their lives, and also pointed to ways in which users can empower themselves to become actors in the change process. Further progress is already being made in some areas, where service users are involved as full participants in the design, delivery and evaluation of their support services. This approach will help to ensure mental health services succeed in supporting local people to achieve their aspirations.

## References

1 Bates P (1996) Stuff as dreams are made on. *Health Service Journal.* **4th April**: 33.
2 Rinaldi M and Hill R (2000) *Insufficient Concern.* Merton Mind, London.
3 Disability Alliance (2005) *The Way to Work – a guide to benefits and tax credits for mental health professionals.* Disability Alliance, London.
4 Department of Health (2002) *Mental Health and Employment in the NHS.* Department of Health, London.
5 Information about the draft Disability Discrimination Bill and about Mind's concerns is available at www.mind.org.uk/News+Policy+Campaigns. Last accessed January 2005.
6 Blackwell T, Burns P and Hard S (2001) *Working Minds: attitudes on mental health in the workplace, with proposals for change.* The Industrial Society, London.
7 OPDM (2004) *Mental Health and Social Exclusion. Social Exclusion Unit report.* Office of the Deputy Prime Minister, London.
8 Clark C, Scott E, Boydell K *et al.* (1999) Effects of client interviewers on client reported satisfaction with mental health services. *Psychiatric Services.* **50**(7): 961–96.

# Chapter 3

# Working wounded

Mo Hutchison

'It's all right Ma, It's life and life only' (Bob Dylan)

Looking back, I can see where it all started to go horribly wrong. I had had a rather troubled childhood: father leaving home, divorce and mother's remarriage contributed in some way to me being a rather insecure and worried teenager – what my mother called 'nervy'. However, I did well at school and college and acquired the necessary 'A' levels to be accepted by universities.

I was to go to Southampton and study psychology. Why psychology? I didn't know. I did know that I didn't want to study anything I had already studied ('A' levels in economics, English and law) but I didn't have a definite career in mind. I hadn't known anyone who had studied psychology. Perhaps it was a presage of things to come. Perhaps I knew at some unconscious level that things psychological were to become a central element of my life.

I enjoyed psychology. I made friends and, in the first term, I met the young man, Paul, who was later to become my husband and, incidentally, contrary to the expressed predictions of some psychiatrists, still is – some 33 years later. However, all was not well. My mind was in constant turmoil. I became obsessed with the suicide of another student and I feared for my own fragile sanity.

Enter my first psychiatrist. A woman with, I was to discover, a Freudian bent who, nevertheless, put me on a cocktail of drugs and ominously warned Paul not to leave me on my own. I think I went out of my mind. It was only with extended stays in the student health centre, and presumably the medication, that I managed to continue having some sort of existence, tortured as that was. I attended few lectures and was able to accomplish very little study but the crucial outcome was that I was establishing the foundations of a career as a mental patient rather than as a graduate social scientist, measuring the components of my life not in promotion and incremental salary increases but in doses of the latest neuroleptics and months between hospital admissions. Yes – that was when things started to go really wrong.

After a traumatic three years, I did obtain a degree. My tutor said that I could have gained a first. In fact, it was a 2:2. I know that, given the severe disruptions and lack of mental acuity, I should have been relieved and even pleased to gain any degree and to an extent I was. But there was still a sense of failure about it, of letting myself down. I did have some ambition relating to research in psychology but I felt this was unlikely to reach fruition as it seemed that to carry out such research, I would need a higher class of degree. Still, I did have Paul, my mainstay.

It is difficult to convey the bizarreness of that time after university. On the one hand I was looking forward to marrying Paul and moving to Liverpool where he was to continue his studies by taking a Postgraduate Certificate in Education. On the other, I was deeply distressed and a week before the wedding I was given a major tranquilliser, stelazine, to help me struggle from one end of the day to the other without too much incident. I was 22 years old and had completely lost sight of the fact that I was on the threshold of a new life where the possibilities should have been thrilling and endless. I just wanted to get by. So much of everyday life had become a challenge. I particularly remember being defeated by a lettuce that needed washing.

We married and after an eventful year in Liverpool, where I first sampled life on an acute psychiatric ward, Paul and I returned south for him to take up a lecturing post in Kent. I also managed to obtain employment using my secretarial qualifications gained at college but my heart wasn't in it and within months I was a patient in one of those monstrous psychiatric institutions which fortunately have largely been consigned to history. (The memory lives on.)

Initially I was there for six months and this was the beginning of a series of admissions each lasting five or six months with little respite between them. In fact, I later wrote that I never really seemed to be discharged but always felt that they were 'keeping my bed warm'. 'The door scarcely had time to close, let alone revolve', I wrote in a letter to *OpenMind*, published by Mind, the National Association for Mental Health in England and Wales.

It was a lonely time. The hospital was remote, Paul was virtually my only visitor and in my early and mid 20s I settled into seeing myself as fatally and irretrievably flawed – one of life's misfits. I was given a handful of drugs, apparently to help me through the day, and another handful to help me through the night. Almost exclusively, my conversations were with those on one side of the mental health divide or the other. I took no interest in events outside the hospital and saw no future for myself in any context outside the psychiatric ward. A move to a long-stay ward was being discussed.

However, one thing that throughout my life has rescued me from some sort of psychiatric oblivion has been the timely intervention of perceptive and caring people. During one admission the ward doctor, recognising that I had a degree in psychology, asked the head of the psychology department if I could help out in the department. Taking some risk, he agreed to a voluntary placement. And so began the process of extending my world beyond the narrow and deranged confines of the ward. Three days a week I left the ward and walked to the psychology department within the grounds of the hospital. There I assisted with testing and research, just like any of the other psychologists, and nobody from outside the department knew any different. I made friends and, wonder of wonders, I was even paid. Not an impressive salary but a few pounds pocket money for which I had to queue once a week in one of the endless corridors along with those also receiving a pittance for sweeping up leaves or whatever. It was a welcome addition to my meagre income. I felt valued as a worker. I was, literally, worth something. It gave a structure to my day and while I was working I seemed to be a different person inhabiting a different world. I was contributing something and though meeting other patients, patients, it has to be said, who were often psychiatrically better off than I was, was scary, I was enjoying the opportunity to be in a psychological environment concentrating on my skills and abilities rather than my weaknesses and disabilities. I was also invited, with Paul, to social events held by members of the department.

There was a downside – I received no support from the ward staff or doctors. It was as though I was doing something vaguely disreputable about which we should not speak. (I don't like to think too much about the ethics of it all and the fact that I had no training whatsoever, otherwise I think I might have concluded that it *was* disreputable!) It was a shadowy existence and my fellow patients on the ward, when they were interested, were bemused by my antics. I don't usually go in for Jekyll and Hyde type analogies but my working role within the department and my sick role within the ward could not have been more different.

In time, my experience in the psychology department allowed me to benefit from a further lucky opportunity. There was another psychiatric hospital about a mile down the road and they had a vacancy for a trainee psychologist they had been trying to fill for some time. To cut a long story short and without even a nod in the direction of equal opportunities, I was appointed to the post and there began an extraordinary period in my life.

In retrospect, I had not really made the transition from patient to worker. In fact, there were times when I was waking up as a patient in hospital A, travelling in the staff bus up the road to hospital B, spending the day there as a basic-grade clinical psychologist and returning to hospital A, and my status as a patient, at the end of my working day. In truth I was hopelessly out of my depth and though I was quite eager to do something vaguely helpful, I had little idea what that might be. Everyone treated me as though I was a qualified clinical psychologist with some years' experience and I did nothing to disabuse them of that view. I also had considerable problems of my own and continued to be maintained on drug doses of biblical proportions.

Once again, apart from my loyal and long-suffering husband, I received no support or supervision. In hospital B, for most of the time I was employed, there was only one legitimate psychologist who was the head of the department. He would arrive for lunch and leave at 3pm. His only contribution to my training was to tell me what an excellent report I wrote – well that's all right then.

I was the only one carrying out assessments or providing any kind of psychological input and I was doing that with the benefit of a few lectures at university and a brief spell as a voluntary worker at hospital A. In my defence, I don't think I actually did anyone any harm but that was probably more by luck than judgement. I was supposed to be training 'on the job' but that training was not provided in the time I was there. The only extension of my education was provided by a short course at the Tavistock Clinic in London on the Rorschach technique (whatever happened to that?). Even when I was living at home, my working life began to mirror the confusion and misery of my personal life and after a year and with little option, I left my job.

During the time I was pretending to be a psychologist, my psychiatrist scarcely alluded to my employment and any problems I might have been having with it, preferring to concentrate on the purely pathological elements of my existence. In fact, of course, they were inextricably entwined.

Some few years on I encountered a psychologist, Tony, who ran a drop-in evening group for people with mental health problems. On occasions I attended this group as an antidote to my extended periods of inactivity broken only by attendance at outpatient appointments. Tony suggested that I apply to a university to register for a higher degree, an MPhil leading to a PhD. I registered at the

City University in London and was accepted in the psychology department to undertake research on my favourite topic, memory. In order to finance my study, I became a nursing assistant working part-time at the local hospital.

Ostensibly my life became more normal and settled. Unfortunately, all was not as it seemed. I was still lacking any supervision or support in either role and my mind was still tormented. I think I considered myself to be a fraud – not quite a doctoral student and not quite a nurse. As far as the nursing was concerned, I was amazed at the responsibilities and duties that nursing assistants were expected to undertake with a couple of weeks training and when someone I was accompanying to the bathroom collapsed and died, my very worst fears were confirmed. I was a liability.

Nevertheless, I did enjoy the extension to my network of friends and colleagues which the university and working as a nurse afforded and when we moved from Surrey to Kent and I was discharged, by default, from the hospital, I began to believe that the course of my life might proceed in a smoother manner. So, despite my misgivings, I continued to work as a nursing assistant and with my research at the university.

However, I was now working on a ward for older people with physical problems and before too long I injured my back while lifting a patient and had to resign. Citing impecunity as the reason, I also informed the university that I could no longer continue my studies. Although this was partly true, I have to admit that I really lacked the confidence necessary to pursue a higher degree. I was forever doubting my abilities and without the benefit of feedback, good or bad, waited with some degree of trepidation to be exposed as the inadequate person I felt myself to be. My guiding motivator was to jump before I was pushed and now I also had a dodgy back to contend with.

From 1977, I assumed a more challenging and rewarding persona – I became a mother – and for a number of years mental health issues couldn't have been further from my mind. Initially I retained my connection with the university and, while pregnant, became a research assistant for the professor of psychology. I continued in this role after my daughter, Jane, was born and as for many mums, the logistics of balancing work and home became a daily challenge. It seemed that I flourished under that type of pressure and when my second child, Tom, was just months old, I became a part-time coordinator of a mental health day centre managed by a local Mind group.

Let me say right away that I do not believe I would have been appointed if there had been any rigorous selection process. There was no application form to be completed, no interview to be undertaken and no gaps in my employment record to be explained. This was before the days of equal opportunities policies and training in selection interviewing and a history of having mental health problems was not seen as a recommendation for any job, particularly not for employment in the mental health field. However, I was appointed and in many ways this became the pinnacle of my achievements. I was able to utilise my burgeoning interest in mental health matters and at the same time received a fairly generous remuneration. My identity became ensconced within a more normal perspective – I was happily married with a nice home, financial security and two fine children. Through my roles as wife, mother and employee, I was able to establish a thriving social and family network and at the same time I was pursuing a stimulating and valued career. Had I finally arrived?

Well, sadly, no I hadn't. Just as this was pre-equal opportunities, it was also a time when little attention was given to the supervisory and support needs of employees, particularly lone workers in stressful working environments. The only occasions I was in a position to receive feedback on my day-to-day activities were when I attended the monthly management committee meetings and these were more about information giving. Although the chair of the management committee called in to see me on a regular if fairly unplanned basis, the meetings were not formal or structured. Tensions between myself and new members of the management committee began to surface, my mental health was suffering and I became distinctly paranoid. My GP thought that I should be referred back to mental health services and, with some misgivings, I suggested that I should visit a psychiatrist I had previously seen who was now a consultant at a London hospital. At the same time I continued to work at the Mind centre and, somewhat to my surprise, found myself pregnant again. Baby Sam arrived and after a short while I returned to work, still with no support, and now Paul and I had three children to organise. It was something of a recipe for disaster and when Sam was just over a year old, disaster did indeed strike. My level of paranoia was rising, I was taking increasing doses of antipsychotics and I was deeply depressed. Hospital was recommended. However, there was a problem as my consultant was in America for the summer and anyway didn't have access to acute beds. With some sleight of hand, I was transferred to another consultant and admission was arranged under his care.

I had told no one at Mind of my mental health difficulties and the chickens were really coming home to roost as I had closed the door on that particular avenue of potential assistance. Much later I was to write an article discussing the pros and cons of disclosure[1] and at the time I believed the following statement: 'Disclosure can be risky because of the degree of stigma and consequent discrimination engendered by the application of a mental health diagnosis'. Accordingly, I informed everyone at Mind that I needed time off to tend a sick relative who lived some distance from me and on the designated day a friend drove me to the hospital in Wimbledon. The image of Paul and the children watching my departure from our front door with tears streaming down their faces is one that will remain with me forever. I had read my Bowlby – what effect was this separation going to have on my family?

The lie about looking after a sick relative became increasingly difficult to sustain as the period of my admission extended from weeks to months and eventually I decided I would have to reveal my secret to the chair of the management committee. She visited me in the hospital and by chance met the registrar who was treating me. She seemed to take an especial interest in his name tag but the significance of that was lost on me at the time.

After three months in hospital I was discharged, still rather troubled and still on high doses of medication. There was no gradual return to work – one day I wasn't there, the next day I was. It was as simple as that. I felt very shaky at work and struggled to maintain an impression of normality. Not only did I feel tremulous, my hands did shake severely as a consequence of the medication I was taking. This embarrassed me and I would go to great lengths not to hold a cup of tea or anything that would reveal it to Mind members. The chair continued to visit me at work from time to time but support was scarce and I only knew that she was concerned about my performance at work when the registrar at the hospital contacted me to say that she had rung him (ah, that's why she made a note of his name), apparently expressing the view that I was too ill to work. Thankfully, the registrar refused to engage in any discussion about me without my knowledge or presence. I lost any trust I might have had in the chair but was determined to keep working.

Gradually my life became a little easier; my children were a delight to me, Paul and I were close and Mind appointed an assistant for me. It seemed that I had emerged from this particular sticky patch relatively unscathed and having partially disclosed my mental health difficulties. It was time to move on. My ambition resurfaced and I applied for a full-time development post with one of the Mind regional offices. This was 1987 and the advertisement for the post was breaking new ground in stating that people who used mental health services were encouraged to apply. Equal opportunity policies were now the norm, as was selection interviewing that concentrated on aptitude, experiences and transferable skills rather than emphasising a chronologically intact employment record and unsubstantiated judgements about suitability. I completed the application form honestly (well, almost), admitting that I had mental health problems that had necessitated admission to psychiatric wards on several occasions. I'm not sure that I detailed exactly how many admissions it had been.

These were still uncertain times and progressive resolve was being tested. I was interviewed for the post and, for the first time, was appointed on my own merits rather than the dubious wheeling and dealing that had preceded my previous jobs. It seemed to me that the time had come to stand up and be counted if we were ever to change the situation of people with mental health problems and the stigma that attached to them. For this reason, prior to leaving the Mind day centre, I informed all members of my past difficulties and my belief that disclosure was the only way of combating discrimination.

Once again I enjoyed a period of relative tranquillity but I have found it pays never to take that at face value as it is often the precursor of more stressful times. After just over two years' employment at the Mind regional office, I found myself needing to use mental health services again. As I knew many mental health professionals within my local area, my GP agreed to refer me to a psychiatrist who practised in the neighbouring town and was recommended by a community psychiatric nurse I knew. From the moment we met he was keen to admit me to his ward but it was several months before I would agree to this course of action and only then because I had lost the ability to make it through each day without incident. His ward was part of a relatively modern mental health unit within the confines of a general hospital. However, it was half an hour's drive from where I lived, posing a problem for family visiting but although it distressed all of us, admission to the unit seemed the only possible solution at the time.

On this occasion there was no need to enter into any kind of subterfuge and I informed Mind about my situation, though I don't think anyone thought that it was as significant as it was to become: not only was I detained compulsorily under the Mental Health Act but I remained an inpatient for over six months. I was also prescribed an array of medication in dizzying proportions.

My immediate line manager visited me in hospital and I agreed that my psychiatrist could be contacted by Mind before I returned to work. As my position within Mind was in a developmental capacity, I recall that my psychiatrist recommended that I should work on small discrete projects where the outcomes could be clearly and quickly seen. Though I'm sure my employers were sympathetic to this viewpoint, it didn't happen and within a relatively short time after discharge I again became completely immersed in the workings of a busy project office.

This was not a good period of my life and for several subsequent years I spent six months at home and six months in hospital. It has to be said that my employers made some attempt to acknowledge the difficulties I experienced in the mornings because of the diurnal variations in my mental health problems and the amount of medication I was taking, and for a while on my various returns to work I was able to work flexitime. Nevertheless, the impact on my personal and working lives was enormous and at one point Mind intimated that they would not renew my contract. The union became involved and the threat was later withdrawn but I knew I was on dodgy ground. I felt pressurised by health professionals to be in hospital and pressurised by my employers to be back at work. That particular conundrum was resolved when, after nine years, funding was withdrawn from the Mind project and I became unemployed. I did also wonder whether I had in fact become unemployable.

After some cajoling from friends and colleagues I compiled a CV which I distributed to various organisations, seeking freelance work. However, before I had received any responses to my request, I was once more admitted to hospital and was again detained, this time for six months. Although I no longer had work to worry about, unemployment had brought financial difficulties which themselves threatened to overwhelm me.

During my stay in hospital, though, I was contacted by the Centre for Mental Health Services Development, then at King's College London, and offered the opportunity to apply to become a freelance associate consultant. I was interviewed and duly appointed to a position as a user consultant where my use of mental health services was not only an asset but a positive requirement – wow! After just over a year I successfully applied for the post of Senior User Consultant, a part-time post (I had to acknowledge that I could not work full time) which I held for five years until July 2003.

During that time I had two more admissions to hospital each for over six months but I dealt with these rather differently, especially the last admission in 2001–2. I later wrote: 'Within a culture of acceptance it is much easier to gather one's strength and make moves in the direction of returning to work,[2] and that was what I did. Having been an inpatient for over two months I began to attend the odd meeting in London to 'keep my hand in' and remind people that I was still around. In fact, I sent regular bulletins from my hospital bed and some work colleagues had visited me there but I still considered that I needed to put in an appearance at King's College. I'm not sure that the strategy was entirely successful as I felt I didn't contribute much to the meetings I attended and I found the whole experience very exhausting, but it did give me a sense of achievement and, I believe, prevented me from further slipping into a substantial lethargy that I feared would overwhelm me.

I am now employed by a national organisation in a role that required not only experience of using mental health services but specifically admission to a psychiatric ward during the previous two years. I am still in touch with mental health services myself and know that admission may, as always, be only a phone call away, but I feel stronger and gratified that those apparently wasted years languishing on psychiatric wards are at long last being put to some good use.

The fact that admission to an acute psychiatric ward had been an essential criterion of my post paved the way for me to include that information in the spiel I gave to the service users I was to interview. I consider this to be empowering. It encourages honesty, the defining of perspective. People knew where I was coming from and related to me in a peer capacity.

In addition, it gave permission for me to create a space within my working life to look after my mental health rather than shut it in the cupboard with the other skeletons (such as they are!). This has been translated into the development of a very supportive relationship with my immediate manager and, indeed, with her manager. Although my mental health is on the agenda it is not in any 'big brother' sense, but rather 'if you need us we're here', even to the extent of having contingency plans for the work to be carried out should I need to be hospitalised again. That is so comforting and reassuring as it removes the pressure on me to keep going no matter what. A pressure that, it has to be said, is in the main self-generated.

I never say, or even think, that if I can overcome the obstacles involved in having a diagnosis of mental illness, so can anyone else. Obviously, there are the interactions of many other variables at play. However, some service users have found my current situation encouraging and, without wishing to overstate it, have sometimes cast me in the position of role model. This is empowering of itself and it humbles me to realise that my achievements are something others would wish to emulate.

So what does work mean to me? It means the opportunity to use the skills I possess. It adds to my personal satisfaction. It gives me a reasonable income. It extends my social network. It allows me to take an interest in other people, other things. It gives me a reason to get up in the mornings, a structure to my days. It makes me a more interesting person. It helps me to feel fulfilled. It contributes to my sense of identity. And so on.

What helps people with mental health problems to obtain and maintain employment? It is my belief, in common with many other service users, that people should be viewed in a holistic way with their mental health problems seen within the broader context of their whole lives, including employment, rather than within the narrow confines of a purely medical approach that often concentrates on weakness and disability rather than strengths and abilities. Nowadays my psychiatrist and psychologist are eager to discuss my employment situation with me, particularly how I can manage this to prevent an exacerbation of my mental health problems. This has been a very helpful strategy, particularly when I have been an inpatient and needed to agree a staggered return to work, but also on a day-to-day basis.

If service users are to juggle with mental health problems and employment successfully, the key requirement would seem to be for them to receive support and that has certainly been lacking until fairly recently in my own experiences. That support can come from a variety of sources: other employees or employers (if the disclosure question has been settled), specialist services designed to help people with mental health problems return to work, mental health services themselves and/or informally from friends and family. In addition, I do consider that it is important for service users to avail themselves of any 'reasonable adjustments' under the UK Disability Discrimination Act of 1995 that could be instituted to make it easier for them to carry out a job. In my own case working from home is much easier, as is starting work later in the morning. Good employment practice is obviously to be recommended: adequate supervision, appropriate training, regular appraisals, anything that reduces stress at work.

This has not always been an easy road to travel. That I have continued to do so is in part due to being in the right place at the right time. It is also, though, testament to the temerity of some employers, to the perspicacity of some mental health professionals, to a tide that is very slowly beginning to turn in favour of those of us with mental health problems who are able to demand something more than pills, poverty and prejudice, to the support and loyalty of my many friends, and to the love, devotion and steadfast belief in me displayed by my family, Paul, Jane, Tom and Sam. It is to these fine people, particularly my family, that this chapter is dedicated.

## References

1  Hutchison M and Nettle M (2001) Deciding about disclosure. *A Life in the Day.* **5**(3): 30–2.
2  Hutchison M (2002) Bridging those troubled waters. *A Life in the Day.* **6**(2): 4–6.

# Chapter 4

# What's kept me working?

Mary Nettle

The best way for me to answer that question is to explain my journey through the mental health system and the ways in which that journey has been linked with work. When I entered the mental health system in the late 1970s, I was in full-time paid work in London as a market research executive for a well-known manufacturer of breakfast cereals. My entry into the system was triggered by my work situation. There had been restructuring and redundancies, which had resulted in many of my colleagues, who were also my friends, losing their jobs. I kept my job but felt I was expected to pick up a lot of their work. I had just got married and had a stressful journey to work in an unreliable car. One day I was asked to produce some figures that had been requested several weeks before. This routine request was the straw that broke the camel's back and I had a hysterical breakdown there and then. I was taken to the factory nurse and did not even know my own name. After several hours and many cups of tea, I had regained my composure and my husband was sent for to take me home. I never went back to that office again.

After some time on Valium, prescribed for me by my GP, I became a zombie, incapable of anything, and was admitted to one of the old asylums. Many things happened whilst I was there but work simply wasn't on the agenda. Although it is a long time ago now, I have a distinct impression that women going out to work was not something that was encouraged. The attitude seemed to be that as I was newly married I should be at home having babies and that this would solve all my problems. I do remember being taken in my drugged-up state to an enormous lecture hall where members of the audience asked me questions about the circumstances of my breakdown. My medical notes were lost with the closure of the hospital and I was never given any information about what was going on, but if memory serves, I think this must have been a conference about the negative impact on women of executive-level work. The occasion itself is certainly a very vivid memory.

After three months I left hospital carrying the label of manic depression, now known as bipolar disorder, and decided to resign from my job. This was partly because I was too embarrassed to go back but also my confidence in my own ability to do a good job had been severely dented. However, a previous employer at a market research agency heard of my situation and offered me a job. Even better, I could start when I wanted to and do a clerical job at an executive salary until I felt able to take up the reins again. This gave my dented confidence a great boost and I went back to work.

However, my husband found a new job in Cirencester and I had to leave my job in London to join him. I applied for a market research executive job in Swindon and after a successful interview, I was sent a letter offering me the job and asking me to attend a routine medical. I attended the medical and was open about my past mental health problems. I then received a letter withdrawing the job offer. The person who offered me the job was mortified but unable to do anything about it. He told me the reason was that the job was felt to be too stressful for me. Hopefully, with the introduction of the Disability Discrimination Act, this scenario can no longer happen but maybe it is just not quite so blatant.

I then applied for a temporary job covering for somebody on sick leave. This time it was not commercial work or market research but part-time work as a clerk at the local cottage hospital. This was a wonderful job. I was taken under the wing of the nurses and the cook and felt part of a big family. I had had an informal interview and no medical was mentioned, as it was only temporary employment. Other service users have said to me they like temping because there is no medical involved. But of course, I had to leave this gentle supportive job when the incumbent returned to work.

At the time, the Royal Air Force base in my town was reopening to support the United States Airforce Europe (USAFE) mission to save the world under President Reagan and I applied for one of the many jobs available as a civilian in the Ministry of Defence. I was successful at interview even though I was open about my mental health problems. One of the people on the interview panel had a daughter who went to the same boarding school as I had and I suspect this overcame any other prejudice the panel might have had. The security checks took a long time but eventually I joined the Morale Welfare and Recreation Department (MWR) and helped set up the base lending library.

I should have realised that I was too independent minded to be a civil servant. I was working on my own when I set up the library but when a librarian from the USA was appointed as my boss, I got a shock: I was expected to type. All American civil servants were able to type and it was an essential requirement for the job. I could use two fingers but this was not good enough and typewriters were not as forgiving as computers – no delete button, just liquid paper in a bottle with a very strong smell. I also had to file according to a manual that made no sense to me; every piece of paper had to be allocated a code and regular filing inspections were undertaken. This was all very stressful. My husband saw the warning signs and persuaded me to visit the GP. I was referred to a psychiatrist who encouraged me to have a stay in hospital. Being a civil servant was not for me and I resigned.

I then began the longest part of this journey, this time as a passive recipient of services and as a volunteer. I had not given up the vision of paid work entirely but I knew I would have to find a way of working that suited me and from which I would not be blocked by prejudice. This was brought home to me when, after several years attending and working as a volunteer driver in the local day centre, I applied to be an occupational therapy helper at the local hospital. I knew one of the occupational therapists there and she had encouraged me to apply. My temporary job at the cottage hospital had been with the same NHS trust so I was surprised after interview to be asked to attend for a medical at the occupational health department as I naively assumed they would know my work history. Needless to say, they concluded that I was mentally unstable and therefore not suitable for the job. This prejudice within the health service against employing people with mental health problems has now been addressed by the Department of Health[1] and some mental health NHS trusts are now beginning to acknowledge that people who have experienced mental ill health, far from being a liability, are likely to be empathetic, highly valued employees. For those trusts that still need convincing, at South West London and St George's Mental Health NHS Trust, 100 people, 41 of whom have a diagnosis of schizophrenia or bipolar disorder, were appointed to both clinical and non-clinical posts between 1995 and 2003 and their sickness absence rates are 3.8% lower than for all other employees. (*See* Chapters 9 and 15 for more about what has been achieved at this trust and some tips on how they have done it.)

Returning to my own journey, I spent the next few years swallowing medication and occupying my time mainly in the garden and about the house. I was an active member of the Women's Institute in my local village too and took part in many village activities. I was also still attending the day centre and one day I was shown a leaflet about an organisation called Survivors Speak Out, which included an invitation to their first conference in Derbyshire. I made contact and went in a minibus with a wonderful bunch of people from Bristol who stopped to pick me up on their way up north. Attending this event was a turning point for me and for many others who went. My eyes were opened to the fact that there was much more to life than being a passive recipient of services. That it was OK to have opinions and that unless you voiced them, nothing would change and services would always be the same.

The next part of my journey still involved volunteering but now it was helping Mind, the national mental health voluntary organisation, to establish Mindlink, the user voice within the organisation. The work meant train journeys to London, conferences in Bournemouth, Brighton, Blackpool and Scarborough and meetings all over the area I was trying to represent, the South West of England. With the support of my peers, my confidence grew and I had almost entered the real world again. But there was one more hurdle to cross – being paid for what I do. This is the barrier at which many people with mental health problems freeze and give up when they are faced with losing the certainty of having the rent paid and a few pounds to live on courtesy of the complex and challenging welfare benefits system.

So how did I make the leap back into paid work? In one way it was easier for me, because I had never been able to claim benefits in the first place. My husband had a highly paid job and I was not eligible for benefits as I was expected to be dependent on him. On the other hand, weaning myself away from my dependency on him for financial support was another turning point for me. At this point in my journey I found myself talking on a train to a fellow service user who had become self-employed as a trainer and consultant. Although she has a PhD and I don't, I do have a Higher National Diploma in Business Studies, a Postgraduate Diploma in Advanced Marketing and several years' practical experience in marketing research. My colleague assured me that I had all the skills required to do what she did and that there was a great demand for those skills. In any case, she argued, we should be paid for what we do. The clincher for me was when she said she would help me. She became what I now would call my mentor and I think this is vital for anyone setting out into paid employment. You need a role model: someone who has been there, done it and got the T shirt; someone who is willing to show you the way and can help you believe in yourself.

Now my journey continued with an ascent into the world of self-employment. I would suggest that people who want to tread this path should take advantage of the opportunities that are on offer from what in my day were called Training and Enterprise Councils and are now called Business Link. I was introduced to a women's officer whose job was to encourage women to take up self-employment. When I told her my idea of becoming a mental health user consultant paid to effect change in mental health services, she was very enthusiastic. I would have to produce a business plan but she offered help with that and there were also courses to attend. Once I had done that, I would be eligible for what was then called the Enterprise Allowance, amounting to £50 a week for a year. Although the allowance is no longer available, an initiative called Business Start Up encompassing many different schemes is available via JobCentre Plus. At the time, Enterprise Allowance was an offer I could not refuse and I became officially self-employed.

In order to ask for money for what you do, you need to value yourself and believe that what you have to offer is of value to other people. The mental health system is very good at devaluing you. You are given a mental illness label, called a long-term patient and considered a victim of your illness. This may be with the best of intentions but it does not help you to value yourself. You need to be aware that you may be ill but that this is a small part of you and you are well able to achieve your aims given the right help and support. When you enter the mental health system for the first time you are likely to be employed, but mental health professionals rarely help you talk to your employer about how you can be helped back to work once you have recovered. The job retention service described in Chapter 14 is an excellent illustration of how valuable that help can be when it is offered.

I have been self-employed for over 10 years now and it is still difficult to ask for money for what I do. Of course, it does get easier and people are far more willing to offer to pay me. This is partly because the climate has changed. User involvement in service development is now expected and accepted, as is the fact that I can expect to be paid like any other consultant. Of course, the rate is lower as it is considered more a vocation than a job!

What has helped me to keep working has been above all peer support from my fellow service users – without them I could not have done it. I feel part of a large family and though I do not often call on their support, I know it's there if I need it. It is like having a big blanket wrapped around you. The use of email and the Internet has been a great help in keeping in touch and providing information without which I would not be able to do the job I do.

For some, having a good home life helps. My own husband died from cirrhosis of the liver after a long descent into alcoholism, but in some ways his inability to be supportive encouraged me to find support from others, so he did me no bad favour by forcing me to broaden my horizons.

I do need supportive professional help from the mental health services and primary care, although I have ongoing battles with them over medication. I would rather not take any but the professionals feel it is too risky for me to stop. Both they and my family feel far more comfortable when I am swallowing the pills. The main thing is I can have a dialogue with them now and they seem to take me seriously. This is a great step forward and long may it continue.

Being self-employed has on the whole been good for my mental health. I am in control and to a large extent I can set my own deadlines. I do not have to earn a lot of money and on the whole it is up to me what goes into my bank account. I can take days off at my convenience and I can work at times of the day that suit me. Email has proved a blessing in that I can communicate with people whenever I like without disturbing them with a phone call or waiting for the post to deliver messages. I like sitting in my dressing gown opening my post and knowing I am at work. I can read reports in the garden and when I get around to investing in a laptop computer, I will be able to write in the garden as well.

There are downsides but with time I have learnt to ignore them or find ways around them. Most work is one-off or short term and there is always the fear that the work will dry up. You have to be proactive and put your name down for conferences so that people are reminded of your existence. The value of networking cannot be overestimated. Although people who know me say this is nonsense, I'm convinced having a memorable surname, Nettle rather than Smith, helps. I also recommend applying, as I have, for posts such as being a Mental Health Act commissioner or a healthcare commission inspector. These provide work for up to 30 days a year and as well as allaying the fear of having no work at all, they also help me to get other work. You need to weave yourself a comfort blanket otherwise the fear of no money coming in can undermine your confidence and in turn decrease your chances of getting work.

Voluntary work as chair or trustee of a charity also can help with contacts and skills, though it is important not to let it take over your life. You still need to earn money and trustees usually cannot be paid. Learning how to say 'no' is hard but must be done. If you have the chance of paid work, take it and do not feel guilty about leaving the voluntary work to later – easier said than done but each time gets easier and people will respect you for it, I hope.

As I have grown older I have become more assertive and more comfortable about valuing my achievements and myself but I still need reassurance that I am doing the right thing. None of the things I have talked about are unique to mental health service users. We all want to be admired and respected and valued for what we do. But the stigma and discrimination that come with using mental health services and having a mental illness label somehow seem to mean we should be treated differently. We do not want to be treated differently. We want to be treated as human beings both inside and outside the world of work.

## Reference

1 Department of Health (2002) *Mental Health and Employment in the NHS*. Department of Health, London.

# Part 2

# Hitting the bottom and getting back up

# Chapter 5

# Getting back to work: what do we know about what works?

Justine Schneider

## Introduction

Like other psychosocial interventions, employment interventions are largely context specific. There are many other factors that affect whether people with mental health problems are able to get back to work and no specific intervention can be implemented or evaluated without taking these into consideration. They include a country's system of healthcare insurance, the incentives or disincentives of welfare benefits, the prevailing labour market, the social stigma associated with unemployment and fears surrounding mental illness, the legislation affecting employers and their respective insurers, and any governmental policies or interventions meant to influence these factors. Such factors will vary from country to country and may create more or less favourable contexts for people with mental health problems to work. This in turn will determine how far effectiveness in one country or context can be translated to another setting where different factors operate.

A burgeoning research literature on vocational rehabilitation over the past years reflects a great deal of investment in development and evaluation in the USA. With a population about 7.5 times that of the UK, the US has both a federal system of vocational rehabilitation and a diverse array of state and local models. Over the past 25 years, studies have supplied a great deal of information about what works or doesn't work in enabling people to get back to work. In making inferences from these data, it is important to bear in mind the particular characteristics of mental healthcare and employment in the United States and how these might impact on the viability of occupational services or the costs and outcomes of those services.

Our aim in this chapter is to review the research literature, giving due weight to evidence from authoritative and systematic reviews but also including some relatively well-contextualised information from other studies of occupational interventions in mental healthcare. We therefore give some space to descriptive and evaluative studies that can help us to understand more fully the range of interventions operating, the variables investigated and the areas where promising results are emerging or where questions remain and further research is indicated. We start by setting out a typology of occupational interventions which, although not uncontroversial, does then enable us to examine the evidence for each type of intervention with some degree of coherence. Having weighed the evidence, we explore the approach that emerges as most effective in more detail and draw conclusions regarding ways forward for both practice and research.

## A typology of occupational interventions

The classification of intervention approaches is crucial to how evidence of effectiveness is interpreted. A vast array of programme labels abounds in the literature, with some programmes having different names for essentially the same approach. A more common occurrence is two programmes with the same label providing very different sets of activities.[1] Informed by our experience of practice in different countries and aware of the broader concerns of mental healthcare providers, we distinguish between three general approaches to occupational interventions for people with mental health problems. One is to provide a work-like setting that is in some way protected or sheltered, a second addresses education or training in the expectation that this will promote employability, while the third aims to help people get real jobs for real pay. We call these sheltered work, training and education, and supported employment. This simplified categorisation can be applied to any country context, although various models operate within each of the three categories.

### Sheltered work

We define sheltered work as any occupational project in which participants, paid or unpaid, have contact mainly with other people with mental health problems and staff members. The category includes four models.

1  Sheltered employment, where people with disabilities or disadvantages are engaged in paid work with other people with disabilities or disadvantages, usually in a protected environment. For instance, hours may be short and transport or meals may be provided.
2  Sheltered workshops, where clients are engaged in work activities in a sheltered setting as above but do not receive a wage at the going rate for the job, although they might receive token or therapeutic payments.
3  Social firms created for the employment of people who are disadvantaged in the labour market and employing at least 30% of employees who fit this description. Related approaches include community businesses (businesses with a legal structure whereby profits are invested in the employees) and cooperatives, a legal structure for companies owned and managed democratically by the employees.
4  Work crews, where small groups of people with disabilities undertake work such as building, decorating or furniture removals.

### Training and education

This category includes interventions that are primarily educational as well as those that are employment-oriented to a greater or lesser degree. What they share is an emphasis on the preparation of the individual. Consequently, they often place less emphasis on employment outcomes than do supported employment interventions. Models within the category include the following.

1 The Clubhouse work-ordered day, by which we mean that element of the Clubhouse model within which members attend as for day care but experience a structured routine designed to facilitate moving onto transitional employment (classed below as supported employment).
2 Rehabilitation/vocational training, where people are taught work-related skills and may obtain formal qualifications. Projects are often located in colleges or training centres and users may undertake unpaid work placements or voluntary work.
3 Supported education, entailing people with expertise in mental health issues advising and supporting people who wish to undertake training and education, either directly or indirectly, through input to the education provider.

## Supported employment

Because wage earning is a critical outcome, this category encompasses all forms of work in open settings for real pay, whether transitional, temporary or permanent. Wage earning sets apart some employment interventions both because of its symbolic significance as evidence of social inclusion and because of its economic impact, permitting the worker to reduce dependency on benefits and become a taxpayer (in principle) or a net contributor to society. Models include the following.

1 The Individual Placement and Support (IPS) approach to supported employment, which involves working full- or part-time in paid, open employment with support as required from a specialist worker.
2 The Supported Placement Scheme (SPS), Workstep and the Personal Advisor Scheme, all schemes for people with disabilities (including those with mental health problems) funded by the UK Department for Work and Pensions (DWP). They offer placement in open employment with some training and support and are provided and monitored by contractors outside the DWP.
3 Clubhouse transitional employment, providing time-limited exposure to open employment, with 'ownership' of the job vested in the Clubhouse, thus freeing the service user from the commitment of taking on the work full-time.
4 User employment, entailing positive discrimination by a provider of mental healthcare at the point of recruitment to enable people with personal experience of mental health problems to access any vacancies for which they are qualified. This is combined with specialist support, provided by the employer.

Inevitably our three categories are open to debate. For example, we have distinguished between two functions of the Clubhouse model: the work-ordered day and transitional employment. Transitional employment is included as supported employment because it does mean people are placed in real jobs for real pay. However, these placements are normally temporary and the job is owned by the Clubhouse, not by the individual, as some definitions of supported employment stipulate.[2] On the other hand, transitional employment is not unlike working for an agency that supplies temporary staff, in this case the agency being the Clubhouse.

The categorisation of social firms and consumer-run enterprises as sheltered work may also be controversial. The rationale here is that these models are at present somewhat segregated from the competitive labour market. They do not usually recruit from the general workforce and they have a relatively high proportion of disabled workers or trainees. Like some other sheltered work settings, social firms participate in the open economy through the sale of goods and services. Social Firms UK, the umbrella body supporting social firm development, makes a clear distinction between economically independent social firms, that employ a mixed workforce where the disabled employees are on the same terms and conditions as everyone else, and sheltered enterprises more akin to day services. However, few such sheltered enterprises manage to become social firms and these, like most sheltered settings, may rely on subsidies, often from mental health service providers, charities or social services. That said, social firms are increasingly located within the social enterprise sector of the economy and while we believe our categorisation is appropriate at the time of writing, in the future it may well be less appropriate. When they do achieve economic independence, social enterprises have considerable potential to provide appropriate supported employment placements for people with mental health problems.

Models also differ in their mode of delivery. In the UK, supported education is likely to be the responsibility of educational providers, while work rehabilitation is likely to be provided by training or rehabilitation experts allied to the health or employment sectors. Each may be delivered in partnership with community mental healthcare providers. Within supported employment, it is recommended that IPS is delivered as an integral part of generic mental health provision, with an employment specialist attending team meetings, having daily contact with the mental health team and participating in decision making.[3] However, IPS has been delivered in specialist services such as assertive community treatment for people with mental health problems who find it difficult to engage with services[4] and early intervention in psychosis services (*see* Chapter 15). Other models of supported employment are delivered by voluntary sector organisations with varying degrees of liaison with mental health services. What is important for our purposes, though, is to focus on the occupational intervention and not to confound this with the mode of delivery or service context.

The evidence for each category of intervention is examined in the following sections of the chapter.

## Sheltered work

Thirteen studies dealing with the outcomes of sheltered work were included in our analysis. One study was excluded because too few people were followed up due to high drop-out rates[5] and one because the groups compared were too different for the comparisons drawn to be valid.[6] Of the 13 studies that were included:

- three were high-quality randomised controlled trials (RCTs)[7,8] or a re-analysis of RCT results[9]

- four were well-designed case control or cohort studies which, though less reliable than RCTs, do provide relatively robust evidence[10–13]
- six were cohort studies from which the evidence is weaker but which are nevertheless informative because they provide information on specific interventions about which little is known, such as social firms.[14–19]

In addition to these 13 studies, we drew on three further papers combining observations with expert opinion that were of theoretical relevance to the topic.[20–22]

## What works or doesn't work?

We found no conclusive evidence that sheltered work of any type is effective in helping people to get back to open employment but we did find evidence of detrimental effects for sheltered workshops.[12, 15] Since throughput rates in these workshops are low and there is some evidence that staff come to perceive users as unable to work, there may be an overall negative effect. Where alternative, more effective provision exists, sheltered work of any kind could arguably reduce the potential for people to obtain open employment by diverting them from more promising intervention models.

## What is promising?

Social firms have the potential to offer individualised and supportive yet socially valued employment and a possible route into open employment for even the most disabled service users. The ratio of non-disabled to disabled workers is critical to the level of social inclusion that they achieve. Not dissimilarly, the non-traditional sheltered employment workshop described by Young[18] may not have better employment outcomes but the ethos of inclusion, if realised, is preferable to the traditional model.

## Training and education

We were unable to include a number of studies examining interventions in this category because the samples researched were highly selective. In addition, the authors provided insufficient information on vocational outcomes, as opposed to short-term direct outcomes of the intervention itself. For example, one RCT looked in detail at training sessions designed to encourage specific career goal orientation and enrolment in education but enrolment was the longest term outcome measured.[23]

Of the 20 studies we were able to include:

- two were high-quality RCTs[24, 25]
- eight were well-designed cohort or case control studies[26–33]
- ten were less reliable but nevertheless informative cohort studies.[12, 15, 34–41]

The interventions studied varied widely, including skills training, work therapy, job finding, psychosocial education and supported education.

## What works or doesn't work?

There is evidence that conventional prevocational training, at least as delivered in the US, is less effective than IPS in terms of employment outcomes. The research also suggests that for education and training approaches to have an impact on employment outcomes, they must have an explicit focus on work, rather than on social skills.

## What is promising?

Cohorts undertaking college- or vocational school-based supported education appear to obtain higher rates of labour force participation than would be predicted for people with severe mental health problems in general, although it is not clear whether there is an interaction with age or diagnosis. This is of particular interest because supported education has been conceived partly in response to the entry-level jobs often gained through supported employment and is designed to enable participants to improve their qualifications in order to get a better job.

The work-ordered day approach of Clubhouses may also offer people the experience or confidence needed to obtain better quality employment, but the overall rates of employment are lower than for supported employment. Moreover, little is known about which components of these Clubhouse programmes lead to good vocational outcomes.

# Supported employment

Supported employment is the approach to occupational intervention that has attracted the most research attention and several previous reviews have been published. However, as Bond and colleagues note,[42] comparisons are often drawn between approaches differing in several ways, leading to alternative interpretations. It is this confusion that we have attempted to avoid by specifying a typology at the outset of this chapter. Of 20 studies included in our analysis:

- two were meta-analyses and one a systematic review of the outcomes of IPS[43–45]
- four were high-quality RCTs[46–49]
- four were less rigorous RCTs[4, 42, 50, 51]
- four were well-designed cohort studies[52–55]
- five were less rigorous but informative cohort or case studies.[56–60]

The two meta-analyses, the systematic review, five of the RCTs and two of the other studies all focus on IPS, as does the one study of user employment where IPS is the model used to support employees.[54] There is therefore a great deal more information about the effectiveness of this model of supported employment compared to any other vocational intervention.

## What works or doesn't work?

All the studies examined conclude that when compared to other vocational interventions, IPS is more effective in enabling people to get real jobs with real wages, even service users who experience multiple disadvantages in addition to their mental health problems. IPS has such unparalleled evidence in its favour that it is now known as evidence-based supported employment. However, none of the most robust evidence comes from a UK context and the quality of the evidence that is available in this context is greatly inferior to that generated in the US.

## What is promising?

It appears that full integration of the IPS model into mental health services promotes its effectiveness. Some work-focused preparation (e.g. induction groups, work readiness training) seems likely to make a difference to job retention.

# Evidence-based supported employment

So what is IPS, what makes it work and how can people with mental health problems be helped to make best use of it?

Although we have described IPS as a 'model' of supported employment for the sake of coherence, the group of US-based researchers most strongly associated with the development and evaluation of IPS do not view it as a distinct model.[1] Rather, they view it as a standardisation of the principles of supported employment, enabling this to be 'clearly described, scientifically studied and implemented in new communities'. To this end they have produced a fidelity scale that assists in standardisation and measurement.[61]

The characteristics of IPS are described as:[62]

1  a clear focus on competitive employment
2  rapid job search
3  integration with mental healthcare
4  responsiveness to user preferences
5  continuous and comprehensive assessment
6  time-unlimited support.

Given that the effectiveness of IPS is well established, researchers have begun to use survey and qualitative methods to explore what makes it work. For example, one study describes how case managers who are more successful in enabling clients to find work are more likely to initiate early discussion about work, deal with clients' fears and raise their aspirations, respond to clients' job preferences, promote disclosure about mental health histories with employers, liaise closely with the employers and remain engaged when a person is in the job.[63]

A second study casts further light on the process of employment support by investigating how work adjustments (termed 'accommodations' in the US) are provided and what areas of functioning – cognitive, social, emotional or phys-ical/other – they address.[64] The authors also measure the frequency of each type of difficulty ('functional limitation'), demonstrating that cognitive imped-iments are most common. These include: learning the job, concentrating, timekeeping, assessing one's own work performance, solving problems/organ-ising work, using language and initiating new tasks. In their study, the number of limitations experienced by individuals bore a direct relationship to the amount of support that they required.

A further study complements this work on limitations by presenting informa-tion about how support has in practice been provided to compensate for individuals' difficulties at work, including low levels of confidence, psychological barriers to particular types of work and the need to learn new skills.[65] The main adjustments required to enable people to live with these difficulties and still do their job revolved around their hours of work, work schedules and job tasks and the authors describe how these were implemented in a number of cases.

Turning to how people can be helped to make best use of evidence-based employment support, there is a long-established body of research around skills training for work, both social skills and work-related skills. In a review of this research, training was found to have a positive effect on skill acquisition and to be associated with a reduction in symptoms but studies rarely examined whether acquired skills were used outside the training setting.[66] Interventions aimed at social functioning alone have seldom been found to improve employ-ment outcomes,[67] a limitation attributed to training being provided prior to job placement and hence outside the appropriate context for learning.[24]

By contrast, Tsang[35] provides some evidence that social skills training in combination with employment support may have a more positive impact. In this study, people receiving social skills training and support into work were more likely to work than a control group at three months' follow-up. Unfortunately, the study did not compare people who received employment support without social skills training to those who received both.

Cognitive difficulties pose problems for people at work, as shown in studies discussed above and elsewhere.[68, 69] An approach that addresses these directly, known as 'errorless learning', is a step-by-step approach to skill acquisition that has its roots in the field of learning disability. Kern and colleagues have found positive results from errorless learning for people with significant cognitive impairment, at least in an experimental setting.[70]

While evidence-based supported employment is demonstrably effective in placing people in employment, it has not always enabled people with mental health problems to retain their jobs for as long as might be hoped. Wallace and colleagues administered a training programme in 'workplace fundamentals' to people with mental health problems who were searching for jobs or recently hired.[33] The content includes: problem identification and problem solving; coping with health issues and drug abuse; interacting with supervisor to obtain feedback; and dealing with setbacks. Particular attention is paid to generalising the lessons learned to real-world settings. The people who completed this train-ing showed superior job retention and higher job satisfaction.[71] Crucially, unlike traditional prevocational training, the timing and focus of workplace skills training involve an actual job, rather than one that is anticipated in the distant future.

These results indicate that training focused on the development and maintenance of workplace skills may be useful as part of the practice of supported employment, at least for some service users. This is not dissimilar to the support currently being offered in the UK as part of the Department for Work and Pension's incapacity benefit reform pilots and the evaluation of those pilots is likely to inform further development of support along these lines.[72] In many respects, such initiatives may be seen as part of the process of accommodation on the part of the employee, mirroring adaptations or adjustments made to the workplace or job. However, this must not obscure the fact that adaptations and adjustments are central to the success of supported employment for many people.

## Conclusions

The research evidence leaves no doubt that Individual Placement and Support, preferably integrated with mental health services, is the way forward in enabling people with mental health problems to get back to work. While the focus must remain on placing and supporting people in real jobs as quickly as possible, errorless learning and workforce skills training, as described above, may support longer term job retention and merit further evaluation as adjuncts to IPS.

Other areas requiring further investigation include:

- whether different types of sheltered work setting, including Clubhouses, encourage service user choice in pathways to employment
- the potential for social firms to create socially inclusive job opportunities for people with high levels of need, with employment support for those who would benefit from this
- the impact of unpaid voluntary work on employment outcomes, since it is widely used and we could find no evidence about its benefits or otherwise
- the provision and employment impact of supported education in the UK context
- in what UK contexts IPS works best, why, for whom and at what cost.

## References

1 Bond G, Vogler K, Resnick S *et al.* (2001) Dimensions of supported employment: factor structure for the IPS fidelity scale. *Journal of Mental Health.* **10**(4): 383–93.
2 Crowther R, Marshall M, Bond G *et al.* (2001) Helping people with severe mental illness to obtain work: systematic review. *British Medical Journal.* **322**: 204–8.
3 Bond G (1998) Vocational rehabilitation. In: R Liberman (ed.) *Handbook of Psychiatric Rehabilitation.* Macmillan, New York.
4 McFarlane W, Dushay R, Deakins S *et al.* (2000) Employment outcomes in family-aided assertive community treatment. *American Journal of Orthopsychiatry.* **70**(2): 203–14.
5 Stein L, Barry K, van Dien G *et al.* (1999) Work and social support: a comparison of consumers who have achieved stability in ACT and clubhouse programs. *Community Mental Health Journal.* **35** (2): 193–200.

6 Knight S and Wishart T (2001) *A Comparison of Employment Initiatives by Three European Partners to Combat the Social Exclusion of Mentally Ill People and their Families.* Department of Health, London.

7 Macias C (2001) *Massachusetts Employment Intervention Demonstration Project. An experimental comparison of PACT and Clubhouse.* Fountain House, New York.

8 Bell M, Lysaker P and Milstein R (1997) Clinical benefits of paid work in schizophrenia. *Schizophrenia Bulletin.* **22:** 51–67.

9 Bond G, Resnick S, Drake R *et al.* (2001) Does competitive employment improve nonvocational outcomes for people with severe mental illness? *Journal of Consulting and Clinical Psychology.* **69**(3)**:** 489–501.

10 Holzner B, Kemmler G and Meise U (1998) The impact of work-related rehabilitation on quality of life of patients with schizophrenia. *Social Psychiatry and Psychiatric Epidemiology.* **33**(12)**:** 624–31.

11 Kates N, Lambrina N, Baillie B *et al.* (1997) An in-home employment program for people with serious mental illness. *Psychiatric Rehabilitation Journal.* **20**(4)**:** 56–60.

12 Reker T and Eikelmann B (1997) Work therapy for schizophrenic patients: results of a 3-year prospective study in Germany. *European Archives of Psychiatry and Clinical Neuroscience.* **247**(6)**:** 314–19.

13 Schultheis A and Bond G (1993) Situational assessment ratings of work behaviours: changes across time and between settings. *Psychosocial Rehabilitation Journal.* 17(2)**:** 107–19.

14 Chan C (2000) *A Multilevel Approach to Supported Employment.* Hong Kong Polytechnic University, Hong Kong.

15 Martin M (1996) Employment rehabilitation schemes for people with mental health problems. *Health and Social Care in the Community.* **4**(5)**:** 271–9.

16 Pannell J, Kandiah R and Summers N (2000) *The Social Firm Initiative.* Bristol Workways Limited and Spectrum Day Services, Bristol.

17 Whittington D (1997) *The Effectiveness of the Industrial Therapy Organisation: The Executive Report on a Three Year Study.* University of Ulster, Ulster.

18 Young K (2001) Working towards recovery in New Hampshire: a study of modernized vocational rehabilitation from the viewpoint of the consumer. *Psychiatric Rehabilitation Journal.* **24**(4)**:** 355–67.

19 Zhang M, Yan H and Phillips M (1994) Community-based psychiatric rehabilitation in Shanghai: facilities, services, outcome and culture-specific characteristics. *British Journal of Psychiatry.* **165**(suppl 24)**:** 70–9.

20 Perkins R (1997) Clubhouses . . . no thanks. *OpenMind.* **88:** 14–15.

21 Nehring J, Hill R and Poole L (1993) *Work, Empowerment and Community.* Research and Development for Psychiatry, London.

22 Pozner A and Jones A (1994) *Outset, Salford: Final Report.* Outset, Salford.

23 Collins M, Bybee D and Mowbray C (1998) Effectiveness of supported education for individuals with psychiatric disabilities: results from an experimental study, *Community Mental Health Journal.* **34**(6)**:** 595–613.

24 Drake R, Becker D, Biesanz J *et al.* (1996) Day treatment versus supported employment for persons with severe mental illness: a replication study. *Psychiatric Services.* **47**(10)**:** 1125–7.

25 Kaufmann C (1995) The self-help-employment-center – some outcomes from the first year. *Psychosocial Rehabilitation Journal.* **18**(4)**:** 145–62.

26 Jacobs H, Wissusik D, Collier R *et al.* (1992) Correlations between psychiatric disabilities and vocational outcome. *Hospital and Community Psychiatry.* **43**(4)**:** 365–9.

27 Bullock W, Ensing D, Alloy V *et al.* (2000) Leadership education: evaluation of a program to promote recovery in persons with psychiatric disability. *Psychiatric Rehabilitation Journal.* **24**: 3–11.

28 Unger K, Anthony W, Sciarappa K *et al.* (1991) A supported education-program for

young-adults with long-term mental-illness. *Hospital and Community Psychiatry.* **42**(8): 838–42.

29 Hoffmann H and Kupper Z (1996) Patient dynamics in early stages of vocational rehabilitation: a pilot study. *Comprehensive Psychiatry.* **37**(3): 216–21.

30 Donnelly M, McGilloway S, Scott D *et al.* (2001) *Vocational Rehabilitation and Training at Action Mental Health: a study of service pathways, programmes and outcomes.* Queen's University Belfast, Faculty of Medicine and Health Sciences, Belfast.

31 Cook J and Solomon M (1993) The community scholar program: an outcome study of supported education for students with severe mental illness. *Psychosocial Rehabilitation Journal.* **17**(1): 83–97.

32 Blankertz L and Robinson S (1996) Adding a vocational focus to mental health rehabilitation. *Psychiatric Services.* **47**: 1216–22.

33 Ellison M, Danley K, Bromberg C *et al.* (1999) Longitudinal outcome of young adults who participated in a psychiatric vocational rehabilitation program. *Psychiatric Rehabilitation Journal.* **22**(4): 337–41.

34 Wallace C, Tauber R and Wilde J (1999) Teaching fundamental workplace skills to persons with serious mental illness. *Psychiatric Services.* **50**(9): 1147–9.

35 Tsang H (2001) Social skills training to help mentally ill persons find and keep a job. *Psychiatric Services.* **52**(7): 891.

36 Klerkz E and van den Bogaard J (2000) Prevocational training in the Netherlands. In: J van den Bogaard (ed.) *Prevocational Training for (ex-)Psychiatric Patients with Abilities in Europe.* ECHO, Jyvaskyla.

37 Mela J and Blasco M (2000) Prevocational training in Catalonia. In: J van den Bogaard (ed.) *Prevocational Training for (ex-) Psychiatric Patients with Abilities in Europe.* ECHO, Jyvaskyla.

38 Monzon E and Vera-Herrera F (2000) Prevocational training in Las Palmas. In: J van den Bogaard (ed.) *Prevocational Training for (ex-) Psychiatric Patients with Abilities in Europe.* ECHO, Jyvaskyla.

39 Van Audenhove C, van Rompaey I and Lissens G (2000) Prevocational training in Flanders. In: J van den Bogaard (ed.) *Prevocational Training for (ex-) Psychiatric Patients with Abilities in Europe.* ECHO, Jyvaskyla.

40 Ahrens C, Frey J and Burke S (1999) An individualised job engagement approach for persons with severe mental illness. *Journal of Rehabilitation.* **65**(4): 17–24.

41 Browne S (1999) Rehabilitation programmes and quality of life in severe mental illness. *International Journal of Social Psychiatry.* **45**(4): 302-9.

42 Bond G, Dietzen L, McGrew J *et al.* (1995) Accelerating entry into supported employment for persons with severe psychiatric disabilities. *Rehabilitation Psychology.* **40**: 91–111.

43 Twamley E, Jeste D and Lehman A (2003) Vocational rehabilitation in schizophrenia and other psychotic disorders: a literature review and meta-analysis of randomized controlled trials. *Journal of Nervous and Mental Disease.* **191**(8): 515–23.

44 Bond G (2004) Supported employment: evidence for an evidence-based practice. *Journal of Psychiatric Rehabilitation.* **27**(4): 345–59.

45 Crowther R and Marshall M (2001) Employment rehabilitation schemes for people with mental health problems in the North West region: service characteristics and utilization. *Journal of Mental Health.* **10**(4): 373–81.

46 McHugo G, Drake R and Becker D (1998) The durability of supported employment effects. *Psychiatric Rehabilitation Journal.* **22**(1): 55–60.

47 Drake R, McHugo G, Bebout R *et al.* (1999) A randomized clinical trial of supported employment for inner-city patients with severe mental disorders. *Archives of General Psychiatry.* **56**(7): 627–33.

48 Lehman A, Goldberg R, McNary S *et al.* (2001) Improving employment outcomes for persons with schizophrenia and other severe and persistent mental illnesses.

*Schizophrenia Research.* **49**: 273–4.

49 Mueser K, Becker D and Wolfe R (2001) Supported employment, job preferences, job tenure and satisfaction. *Journal of Mental Health.* **10**(4): 411–71.

50 Okpaku S, Anderson K, Sibulkin A *et al.* (1997) Effectiveness of multidisciplinary case management intervention on the employment of SSDI applicants and beneficiaries. *Psychiatric Rehabilitation Journal.* **20**(3): 34–41.

51 Bedell J, Draving D, Parrish A *et al.* (1998) A description and comparison of experiences of people with mental disorders in supported employment and paid prevocational training. *Psychiatric Rehabilitation Journal.* **21**: 279–83.

52 Johnson S, Mitchell D and Avis M (2001) *An Analysis of the Costs and Benefits of The New Deal For Disabled People Personal Adviser Service and the Supported Placement Scheme in Shaw Trust Clients. Report prepared for the Shaw Trust.* University of Nottingham, Nottingham.

53 Rogers E, Sciarappa K, MacDonald-Wilson K *et al.* (1995). A benefit-cost analysis of a supported employment model for persons with psychiatric disabilities. *Evaluation and Program Planning.* **18**(2): 105–15.

54 Perkins R, Rinaldi M, Hardisty J *et al.* (2001) *User Employment Programme Progress Report, September 2001.* South West London and St George's Mental Health NHS Trust, London.

55 Drake R, Becker D, Biesanz J *et al.* (1994) Rehabilitative day treatment vs supported employment: 1. Vocational outcomes. *Community Mental Health Journal.* **30**(5): 519.

56 Secker J, Membrey H, Grove B *et al.* (2002) Recovering from illness or recovering your life? Implications of clinical versus social models of recovery from mental illness for employment support services. *Disability and Society.* **17**(4): 403–18.

57 Chandler D, Meisel J, Hu T *et al.* (1997) A capitated model for a cross section of severely mentally ill clients: employment outcomes. *Community Mental Health Journal.* **33**: 501–16.

58 Bailey E (1998) Do long-term day treatment clients benefit from supported employment? *Psychiatric Rehabilitation Journal.* **22**(1): 24–9.

59 Warner R and Polak P (1995) The economic advancement of the mentally ill in the community: 1. Economic opportunities. *Community Mental Health Journal.* **31**(4): 381–96.

60 Seeman M and Seeman B (2000) Earning money via the Internet: perceptions of women with schizophrenia of in-home computer working. *International Journal of Psychosocial Rehabilitation.* **5**: 35–40.

61 Bond G, Evans L, Salyers M *et al.* (2000) Measurement of fidelity in psychiatric rehabilitation. *Mental Health Services Research.* **2**(2): 75–87.

62 Bond G, Drake R, Mueser K *et al.* (1997) An update on supported employment for people with mental illness. *Psychiatric Services.* **48**: 335–46.

63 Gowdy E, Carlson J and Rapp C (2003) Practices differentiating high-performing from low-performing supported employment programs. *Psychiatric Rehabilitation Journal.* **26**: 232–9.

64 MacDonald-Wilson K, Rogers E, Massaro J *et al.* (2002) An investigation of reasonable workplace accommodations for people with psychiatric disabilities. *Community Mental Health Journal.* **38**(1): 35–50.

65 Secker J, Membrey H, Grove B *et al.* (2003) The how and why of workplace adjustments: contextualizing the evidence. *Psychiatric Rehabilitation Journal.* **27**(1): 3–8.

66 Dilk M and Bond G (1996) Meta-analytic evaluation of skills training research for individuals with severe mental illness. *Journal of Consulting and Clinical Psychology.* **64**: 1337–46.

67 Mueser K, Bond G and Drake R (2001) Community-based treatment of schizophrenia and other severe mental disorders: treatment outcomes? *Medscape Mental Health.* **6**:1.

68 Gold J, Goldberg R, McNary S *et al.* (2002) Cognitive correlates of job tenure among patients with severe mental illness. *American Journal of Psychiatry.* **159**: 1395–402.

69 Dickerson F, Boronow J, Stallings C *et al.* (2004) Association between cognitive functioning and employment status of persons with bipolar disorder. *Psychiatric Services.* **55**: 54–8.

70 Kern R, Green M, Mintz J *et al.* (2003) Does 'errorless learning' compensate for neurocognitive impairments in the work rehabilitation of persons with schizophrenia? *Psychological Medicine.* **33**: 433–42.

71 Wallace C and Tauber R (2004) Supplementing supported employment with workplace skills training. *Psychiatric Services.* **55**: 513–15.

72 Department for Work and Pensions (2003) *Pathways to Work: helping people into employment.* The Stationery Office, Norwich.

Chapter 6

# Employment support in the UK: where are we now?

Justine Schneider

## Introduction

Commissioners are under pressure to increase employment opportunities for service users with mental health problems to aid recovery and promote social integration. The Social Exclusion Unit report[1] on employment and mental health advocates the Individual Placement and Support (IPS) approach described in the previous chapter. This chapter presents the results of a survey examining the current operation of supported employment in the UK for people with mental health problems. The survey was part of a wider study of employment support for all disability groups to which 423 employment officers working with people with mental health problems responded.

Respondents were asked to describe their practice using a measure, the Supported Employment Adherence Scale, which we developed for the study along similar lines to the functional analysis produced by Bysshe and colleagues.[2] This differs from the fidelity scale developed by Bond and colleagues[3–6] in that it rates the behaviour of the employment officer, rather than organisational-level features of a service. The adherence scale lists 23 activities derived from the literature and expert opinion to represent the core activities of employment support (Box 6.1).

---

**Box 6.1 Supported employment adherence indicators**

---

Individual counselling about work
Giving careers/training advice
Giving benefits advice
Job/vocational profiling (identifying employment goals and abilities)
Job search training (CV and interview preparation/support)
Job finding and placement/matching jobs to individuals (long term)
Setting up work tasters/trials (short term)
Providing work skills training/social skills training prior to placement
Reviewing and developing clients' jobs
Job coaching or training (in the workplace)
Off-site job support/coaching (away from the workplace)
Co-worker education/counselling
Drawing on and developing 'circles of support'

> **Box 6.1 Supported employment adherence indicators** *(contd)*
>
> Drawing on and developing 'natural supports'
> Responding to supervisors' or employers' concerns about individual clients
> Assessing the accommodations/adaptations needed
> Negotiating/advocating with employers or supervisors on behalf of clients
> Negotiating/advocating on behalf of clients with their co-workers
> Negotiating/advocating with carers on behalf of clients
> Promoting and advocating employment opportunities
> Reviewing/evaluating the effectiveness of employment programmes
> Promoting employer rights and responsibilities
> Promoting the social model of disability.

Information about the employment officers themselves was obtained to illustrate the diverse settings from which employment support may be derived. In addition, they were asked about their client groups and caseload size and were invited to tell us about up to three clients they had most recently placed in jobs, describing the individual and the job itself. The employment officers provided information about 264 recently placed clients whom they judged to have mental health problems.

In the sections that follow we describe the employment officers and their clients and then draw out conclusions about the current stage of development of supported employment in the UK and the further developments required.

## The employment officers

Individual employment officers were promised anonymity but we can say that five or more (at least 1% of the total) worked for the following agencies: Shaw Trust, JobCentre Plus, Remploy, Scope, Mencap, Richmond Fellowship, Support into Work, Co-Options, Oaklea Trust, Employment Opportunities, Action Mental Health, Triangle Housing Association, Hansel Alliance, East Sussex Council and Cheshire Council. In some cases mental health problems may not have been the client's only disability.

The Department for Work and Pensions (DWP) is responsible for the national network of JobCentre Plus services, which was undergoing reorganisation at the time of the survey. As a consequence, only about one-fifth of their disability employment advisors were included, so the proportion of respondents working in JobCentre Plus is an underestimate. Overall, 38% of respondents worked for voluntary organisations, 18% for local authorities, 9.5% for JobCentre Plus and 3% for health providers. Remploy defines itself as a private business and 11.5% of employment officers described themselves in this category. The remainder gave their employer as 'other' (15%) or did not respond (5%).

## Work settings

Table 6.1 shows all the settings in which employment officers for people with mental health problems were working. The largest proportion said their work setting was supported employment (39%) but 20% described their setting as work rehabilitation or training. It is interesting to note that 25% were working in statutory DWP contexts, as Workstep contractors or as part of a disability team in JobCentre Plus. Other people who described themselves as employment officers were found in educational settings, which could also include Connexions, a service for young people in transition from school to further education or employment. Smaller numbers of respondents were in day centres, sheltered employment, social firms and Clubhouses.

**Table 6.1 Settings where respondents were located**

|  | % (*n* = 423) |
|---|---|
| Supported employment | 39 |
| Work rehabilitation/training | 20 |
| Workstep | 15 |
| Disability team – JobCentre Plus | 10 |
| Supported education | 5 |
| Day centre or resource centre | 4 |
| Social firm | 2 |
| Connexions | 2 |
| Sheltered employment | 1 |
| Clubhouse | 0 |
| Missing | 2 |
| Total | 100 |

## Specialist and generic settings

We had complete adherence scale scores for 137 employment officers who told us about one or more recently placed clients. One did not give a setting for their work. We categorised as 'specialist' employment officers the 86 who were in the following settings: Workstep (17), Supported Employment (57) and JobCentre Plus disability teams (12). Box 6.2 shows how we defined 'specialist'. In contrast with the central focus of these specialist settings on real jobs, settings such as day centres and work rehabilitation were categorised as 'generic'.

## Supported employment adherence scores

The mean supported employment adherence score for the employment officers was 67.29 (standard deviation 12.50, range 29–91). Tables 6.2 and 6.3 show the mean scores by agency and work setting. Agencies and settings with sample sizes below five have been omitted from these tables for the sake of reliability. Different sample sizes make it difficult to apply statistical tests but inspection of the tables suggests that the lowest mean adherence scores are found in health agencies and day centre settings. Not surprisingly, the highest scores were in settings offering supported employment, while there is little to choose between the mean adherence scores in voluntary agencies, private businesses, JobCentre Plus and local authorities.

Table 6.2 Mean adherence scale scores by agency

| Agency | Mean | Standard deviation | n |
|---|---|---|---|
| Voluntary organisation | 68.00 | 12.51 | 80 |
| Private business | 66.57 | 8.96 | 7 |
| JobCentre Plus | 66.25 | 10.64 | 12 |
| Health provider | 59.33 | 20.13 | 6 |
| LA – Social Services | 67.86 | 11.77 | 29 |

Table 6.3 Mean adherence scale scores by setting

| Agency | Mean | Standard deviation | n |
|---|---|---|---|
| Work rehabilitation | 65.84 | 14.20 | 38 |
| Day/resource centre | 57.20 | 22.72 | 5 |
| Workstep | 66.41 | 12.93 | 17 |
| Supported employment | 70.37 | 9.81 | 57 |
| Disability team – JobCentre Plus | 65.50 | 11.26 | 12 |

## Focus on mental health

Very few employment officers appeared to focus exclusively on mental health issues. Most worked with other client groups as well (88%), including people with learning disabilities, autistic spectrum disorder, acquired brain injury, physical disabilities and sensory disabilities. A few (7%) also worked with non-disabled people who are not otherwise disadvantaged. Almost all (96%) told us that they had some contact with employers and virtually all (99%) had regular contact with families or carers of the people with whom they worked.

> **Box 6.2 Specialist supported employment: a definition[7]**
>
> A key assumption underlying the specialist sector's approach to supported employment is that the workplace is the best place to learn a job. As a matter of principle, it starts from the assumption that all disabled people may wish to access paid work and that no individual or group should be seen as 'unemployable'. It is concerned with addressing some of the social, attitudinal, policy and practice barriers that exclude groups from paid work.

Box 6.2 Specialist supported employment: a definition[7] *(contd)*

The approach also attempts to set paid work in its wider social context. It is concerned with inclusion, in terms of both economic and social participation; it is meant to be about 'real' jobs in ordinary (non-segregated) workplaces.

Supported employment agencies inevitably vary in their approach (and in the extent to which they are able to put the ideal of supported employment into practice) but typically offer a combination of:

- helping people identify their skills and preferences through the development of a vocational profile
- job development to find the person's preferred job through contact with employers
- job analysis to find out more about the workplace, co-workers and the support the individual might need in that environment
- job support to ensure that both the employee and employer receive 'just enough' creative assistance, information and back-up to achieve success, with this support continuing as long as it is needed
- career support to help people think in the longer term about career progression.

## Qualifications

Thirty-five per cent of respondents had a professional qualification that we judged to be directly relevant to the work of an employment officer, including a qualification in supported employment, counselling, careers guidance, social work, teaching, adult training or occupational therapy. We also counted other professional qualifications, such as nursing and psychology, at any level and degrees in any subject, which applied to a further 25%. Even so, 40% had no relevant qualifications. On average they had worked in their present jobs for four years (range 0–32).

## Caseloads

The mean caseload size was 52 (range 0–932). Given the difficulty of providing a personal service to more than 100 clients, respondents with a caseload larger than this were examined separately. Of the 37 to whom this applied, five were disability employment advisors, five called themselves employment coordinators, five had the word 'manager' in their job titles and two were careers officers. This group of people with large caseloads was therefore taken to have mainly managerial responsibilities. Excluding them, the mean caseload size was 35 (range 0–99) and the mean number of clients from ethnic minorities on these caseloads was three (range 0–50). People with smaller caseloads (defined as 15 clients or fewer) were no more likely to have placed their clients in paid work, as compared to unpaid jobs.

# The clients

Fifty-six per cent of the 264 clients with mental health needs were male, with an average age of 37 (standard deviation 9.92). Because our informants were not clinicians, we have no diagnostic information and no ratings of levels of need for their clients. The information we do have concerns the number of hours employment officers worked with clients prior to placing them in a job, and clients' educational and employment backgrounds.

## *Hours worked with clients before job placement*

Although we have no information about clients' level of need, at face value it might be argued that the amount of time spent with a client before job placement could be taken as one indication of this. The problem with this is that there are also likely to be organisational factors that determine the length of time spent with each client, regardless of needs. One of these factors is the length of set courses of work preparation. A second is financial incentives – for example, Workstep pays the contractor a lump sum for each job start. Another is the orientation of the agency; given that there is evidence to support shorter periods of preparation over longer ones,[8] providers whose input is evidence-based are more likely to offer shorter periods of job preparation.

Table 6.4 indicates that on average, social services worked with their clients for the longest period of time before placement, while health providers worked for the shortest period of time. However, these means were not significantly different because of the variation within each sample and the difference in sample sizes.

**Table 6.4 Mean hours input from employment officer prior to placement**

| Agency | Mean | Standard deviation | $n$ |
| --- | --- | --- | --- |
| Voluntary organisation | 26.92 | 47.93 | 141 |
| Private business/organisation | 21.57 | 46.97 | 7 |
| JobCentre Plus | 13.07 | 12.82 | 15 |
| Health authority | 6.33 | 6.14 | 9 |
| LA – Social Services | 38.90 | 41.47 | 52 |
| Total | 27.78 | 44.39 | 224 |

## *Education and employment*

Forty per cent of those users of employment support for whom data were provided had five or more GCSEs (equivalent to high school diploma or school leaving certificate at age 16) and 79% had prior paid work experience. Precisely half (132) were in paid open employment (unsupported or supported), five were in paid sheltered work and the rest were in training, work experience placements or unpaid, voluntary work.

The jobs clients had obtained had lasted on average four months (range

0–36), but the low mean duration is because employment officers were asked for details of their three most recent placements. About 20% had gone into retail jobs, about 20% into health and social work, with about 10% each in hotels and restaurants, and administrative or clerical work. The numerous jobs described as 'other' were diverse: animal care, cleaning, computer design, hairdressing, teaching, library work, market research, recycling, security and zoo work. Fourteen per cent of the people recently placed were no longer in the job but employment officers were not asked to explain the reasons for this.

## Pay and benefits

Social security benefits are often regarded as a disincentive to paid employment, so we asked which of two key benefits people were receiving. At the time of the survey, entitlement to Income Support was reduced pound for pound if a person earned more than £20 per week, whereas people on Incapacity Benefit could earn up to £72 per week if they were receiving support from mental healthcare providers but were only allowed to work up to 16 hours. We found that 25% of the 264 clients were getting Income Support, 40% were getting Incapacity Benefit, 21% were in receipt of both benefits and 16% were not on any benefit.

The employment officers were asked if the client earned at least the national minimum wage (NMW), which applies to disabled people as well as others. Of the 137 people in paid employment, 130 (95%) were earning at least the NMW. For two people this information was missing but five were not earning the NMW. Two of these people were in sheltered work placement, one was in open employment and two were in supported employment.

# Discussion

The employment officers themselves are our only source for this survey. It was clear early on in the study that they do not work within a medical model and therefore were not likely to respond reliably to questions framed in terms of conventional measures of need or disability. Although this lack of diagnostic data limits the inferences that can be drawn from the survey, the relatively large sample of people with mental health problems in employment, unprecedented in the UK, allows us to describe a reasonably representative cross-section of employment officers and their clients.

Many people with mental health problems receive support into employment from a range of agencies in a number of different settings. The key providers are the large voluntary organisations, the Department for Work and Pensions and local authorities. Health providers are not a major source of employment support for people with mental health problems.

The employment officers supporting people with mental health problems tended to work across disability groups and were not, for the most part, specifically trained in the work that they do. They have a wide range of professional backgrounds but 40% do not claim to have any qualifications relating to supported employment. A typical caseload comprised about 35 individuals.

The amount of time spent preparing a person with mental health problems for work varied according to the agency concerned, with an overall mean of 28 hours' input. This input may depend on the level of need of the person concerned but it may also reflect low expectations on the part of providers about people's ability to move quickly to real jobs. By comparison, the mean time spent preparing a person with a physical disability was significantly shorter at 18 hours.

The work that people with mental health problems obtained was diverse but 84% of them were still receiving Incapacity Benefit or Income Support or both. This may be partly because the placements were recent, so that some people may not yet have made the step to independence from state benefits. It was clear that the small percentage of people who were not getting either of these benefits were more likely to be in paid employment, as compared to voluntary work or training, but this is not a surprising result since people who were not being paid would be unlikely to have any source of income other than benefits.

For people with mental health problems, being placed by an employment officer from a specialist setting (Workstep, JobCentre Plus or a supported employment agency) significantly increased the probability of obtaining paid work. Yet compared to other disability groups, notably people with learning disabilities, people with mental health problems appear to have less access to specialist employment officers. This is likely to have an adverse impact on their probability of obtaining paid employment.

It may be somewhat surprising that, several years after the introduction of the national minimum wage, there are still people who do not earn this minimum income. This reflects enduring confusion about the rules, their applicability to people with disabilities and the fact that employers seem to lack information about how to operate them.[9, 10] Failure to pay the NMW has been recognised as a problem for sheltered workshops since its introduction in 2001, but the number of sites where there is a discrepancy between the NMW and clients' pay is declining as the NMW is increasingly enforced.

## Conclusion

It is evident from our survey that employment support for people with mental health problems is at an early stage of development in the UK and we are clearly some distance from widespread provision of evidence-based supported employment as described in the previous chapter. Issues of particular concern include the following.

- There are very few employment officers working within mental health settings, as recommended by the international evidence.
- Few employment officers specialise in working with people with mental health problems.
- Adherence to effective supported employment indicators is not high, though highest, unsurprisingly, among officers who describe themselves as working in supported employment settings.
- People working in JobCentre Plus, Workstep and supported employment settings had more clients in paid work than those working in day centres or rehabilitation and training settings.

- Average caseloads are considerably higher than the maximum recommended active caseload of 12–15 but clients on small caseloads were no more likely to be in paid work.

Since most support into employment is currently provided outside mental health services, in the short term commissioners may need to harness those services that are available to meet the needs of people with mental health problems. At the same time, however, action is urgently required to ensure that people who need to use mental health services have access to the most effective approaches to employment support. At an organisational level, indications from the US are that these should ideally be fully integrated with mental health services and adhere to the indicators derived from the international evidence base, as encapsulated in the Supported Employment Fidelity Scale.[3–6] As Miles Rinaldi and Rachel Perkins demonstrate in Chapters 9 and 15, this has been achieved in South West London. Where organisational structures are lacking, individual officers' practice may be assessed according to the adherence scale developed for our survey. If the will is there to overcome old ways of thinking about employment and mental health, there is no reason why it cannot be achieved throughout the UK.

# References

1 OPDM (2004) *Mental Health and Social Exclusion. Social Exclusion Unit report.* Office of the Deputy Prime Minister, London.
2 Bysshe S, Bell D and Parsons D (2002) *Employment and Disability Functions in the United Kingdom: an occupational and functional review.* HOST Policy Research, Horsham.
3 Bond G, Becker D, Drake R *et al.* (1997) A fidelity scale for the individual placement and support model of supported employment. *Rehabilitation Counselling Bulletin.* **40**: 265–84.
4 Bond G, Picone J, Mauer B *et al.* (1999) The quality of supported employment implementation scale. In: G Revell, D Mank, P Wehman (eds) *The Impact of Supported Employment for People with Significant Disabilities.* VCU-RRTC on Workplace Supports, Virginia.
5 Bond G, Evans L, Salyers M *et al.* (2000) Measurement of fidelity in psychiatric rehabilitation. *Mental Health Services Research.* **2**(2): 75–87.
6 Bond G, Vogler K, Resnick S *et al.* (2001) Dimensions of supported employment: factor structure for the IPS fidelity scale. *Journal of Mental Health.* **10**(4): 383–93.
7 O'Bryan A, Simons K, Beyer S *et al.* (2000) *A Framework for Supported Employment.* Joseph Rowntree Foundation, York.
8 Bond G, Dietzen L, McGrew J *et al.* (1995) Accelerating entry into supported employment for persons with severe psychiatric disabilities. *Rehabilitation Psychology.* **40**: 91–111.
9 Schneider J, Simons K and Everatt G (2001) Impact of the national minimum wage on disabled people. *Disability and Society.* **16**: 723–47.
10 Schneider J and Dutton J (2002) Attitudes towards disabled staff and the effect of the national minimum wage: a Delphi survey of employers and disability employment advisors. *Disability and Society.* **17**: 283–306.

# Chapter 7

# Recovering a life: an in-depth look at employment support in the UK

Jenny Secker, Bob Grove and Helen Membrey

## Introduction

As Justine Schneider has illustrated in the previous chapter, approaches to providing employment support vary widely in the UK. In this chapter we present the results of a study that explored some of those variations in greater depth. Although small in scale, the study illuminated a clear need for employment support workers and mental health professionals to work far more closely together and for their work to be underpinned by social as opposed to clinical understandings of the processes of recovery from mental ill health. Such is the dominance of the 'illness' model of mental distress that this could prove a tall order, even for non-clinicians.

We wanted to explore approaches to and experiences of employment support from the perspectives of those involved and semi-structured interviews were therefore chosen to carry out the research. Five projects providing specialist employment support to people who had experienced mental health problems offered to help with the study. Four of the projects operated within the voluntary sector, while the fifth was established by a local authority social services department. With the assistance of the five projects, 17 clients who had been placed in open employment were contacted and agreed to be interviewed. Eleven clients had been able to retain their job for 12 months or longer. The jobs of the other six clients had broken down within 12 months, usually within a matter of weeks. All 17 clients gave permission for their employment project worker and workplace manager to be interviewed and a total of 51 interviews were carried out.

Analysis of the interviews resulted in the construction of a framework within which the retention or breakdown of clients' jobs could be understood. The framework encompassed a continuum of approaches to employment support, with two projects, described here as Projects A and D, at the extremes of the continuum. Because these two projects exemplified the greatest variation in approach, we focus largely on those projects here, although our analysis is informed by all 17 cases studied. In presenting the results of the study, we describe the different approaches to employment support at Projects A and D, draw out the underlying models of recovery implicit within the two approaches and consider their relative strengths and limitations. Following a discussion of their implications of the results, we put forward conclusions regarding the future development of employment support in the UK.

## The projects' approaches to employment support

A total of seven cases were studied from the two projects, four from Project A and three from Project D. Of the seven clients concerned, five had been able to retain their job for 12 months or longer while two, both from Project A, had experienced the breakdown of their job within a matter of weeks. The approach taken to employment support at each project is described in turn below in relation to assessment, job preparation, job finding and support in work.

### Project A

In terms of assessment and job preparation, a two-tier approach was in place at Project A, reflecting an expectation that to embark on paid employment, clients should have recovered from their mental health problems or at least be more or less symptom free, if necessary with the aid of medication. When new clients were referred to the project, an initial interview was carried out to assess whether the client had recovered sufficiently to move straight to job finding or whether job preparation was required.

When a client was assessed as already sufficiently recovered, further assessment or job preparation was seen as unnecessary and the client's mental health problems were not seen as having implications for work. Instead, the focus was on how readily they would fit into and function in the world of work.

> I think we have an unwritten policy of taking people at face value. So if someone comes along and wants to work, get to know them, find out what they want to do and give them an opportunity, rather than dwell on anything else that might be going on. Obviously you are aware of it but in a kind of real work situation it's who turns up at nine in the morning that has the job. It's not the baggage they've got with them.

The assistance provided for these clients consisted of an invitation to attend a job club, held on one morning each week, where information about vacancies was made available. Although help with the application process was provided if required, project workers did not see it as part of their role to explore clients' career options with them in any detail or assist them in pursuing their goals.

When new clients were thought to require job preparation, the emphasis was on using this period of 'convalescence' to bring their skills up to scratch through a structured training course and to develop the stamina required to cope with work through an unpaid work placement, usually six weeks in length. Although it was hoped in some cases that an unpaid placement might lead to paid work, as with clients who were assessed as ready for work on referral, project workers did not see it as their role to help with this.

> We don't find patients employment, we let them find their own. The idea is they find employment, we support them in every way possible, they're getting the confidence, getting stamina back and getting a job is a bonus as we see it. But the patient has to find it themselves.

Equally, in identifying placements, workers did not seek to pursue clients' individual career goals. Instead, the project relied on an established pool of employers, allocating placements on the basis of what was available, coupled with an assessment of whether clients would fit in at that workplace. Once a potential placement had been identified, an interview was arranged and a project worker would accompany the client to the interview. However, it was regarded as the responsibility of the client to let the employer know of any needs they might have. In this respect, the project worker's role was seen as that of an 'introducer', as one workplace manager put it, and identifying and resolving any potential problems was not part of the process of negotiating a placement. What was important, from the project workers' point of view, was that the employer should feel confident that their own needs would be met, in terms of the client's capacity to do the work required.

Once an unpaid placement had been set up for a client, the system for providing support consisted of visits to the placement every two weeks, with a formal review after six weeks. From the workers' accounts, the two-weekly visits were fairly informal, involving a brief discussion with the client followed by a separate meeting with the manager. As at the stage when placements were being set up, the focus remained on how well the client was doing the job required by the employer.

> It's just to see how things are going, just sit down with [the client] and have a general chat... and then I would have a chat with [the manager]... and we ask employers to be honest as well. We don't want them saying they feel sorry for the client, we want them to be honest here; if he's not doing the work, say so.

Because the visits involved separate discussions with the client and manager, there was no opportunity for clients to discuss their needs with managers or for managers to provide feedback to clients. At the six-week review, however, the project worker, client and manager did meet together to discuss the placement and the manager, but not the client, was asked to complete a review form. Here again, then, the focus appeared to be more on the client's performance in the job than on their needs, an impression supported by this manager's recollection.

> I think it was pretty much [the project worker] asking the odd question but me and [the client] talking directly... how am I doing, how quick am I working, you know, am I making the grade sort of thing. It was more to do with on-the-job kind of stuff than where [the project worker] was coming from.

Once clients were in paid work, contact with the project was minimal and workers had no contact with clients' workplaces unless they were requested to do so by clients. The arrangement for clients was that they should drop into the job club or contact the project for an appointment during job club hours if they wanted to discuss any concerns, and contact outside these hours was discouraged. As this project worker indicated, the provision of follow-up support in paid work was antithetical to the project's equation of readiness to work with recovery from illness.

> It's not fair to clients to be in contact. If they're working they've left
> their illness behind them... they don't want us going in and visiting
> and talking to the employer.

## Project D

A first indication of the different approach taken at Project D was an assumption that all clients would need a period of assessment and job preparation. The
three clients interviewed from the project had all been involved with the project
for over a year before starting work and workers at Project D did not describe
other cases where clients had moved straight into work. In contrast, all four
clients from Project A had obtained paid work within two months or less.

The assumption that clients would need a period of assessment and preparation stemmed from a view that construed mental health problems not as an
illness from which people needed to recover in the clinical sense before working
but as an intrinsic aspect of a client's life experience that had implications for
work.

> You need to talk with the individual, to start identifying how their
> particular illness affects them ... and that can be simple things like,
> what's the best time of day for you, when does the medication kick
> in?

In accordance with this stance, workers at Project D made extensive use of individual interviews, not to assess clients' ability to fit into the world of work but
to understand, and enable the client to understand, the career options and type
of workplace that might best suit them and to address specific psychological
barriers to work. Although assessment and job preparation were therefore
intensive at Project D, this was seen only as a step along the way, to be built on
once clients were in work. At this project, the emphasis in job finding was on
negotiating work trials for clients in the explicit expectation that, if the trial
were successful, paid work would result. In keeping with the focus of assessment and job preparation on their particular needs, clients were not expected
to fit in with what was available. Although the project did have a pool of known
employers, a client would not be placed with an employer unless the worker
was convinced the job was appropriate for that client.

This attention to clients' needs was also evident in the way in which work
trials were negotiated with employers. At Project D, it was standard practice for
workers to accompany clients to interviews in order to ensure that the client's
needs would be met. However, employers' needs were also recognised, not only
in terms of the client's ability to do the job but in terms of the manager's own
support needs.

At Project D, workers also saw providing ongoing support to clients as a
central role, both during their work trial and once they were in paid work. As
with work experience placements at Project A, the support provided consisted
of informal contact combined with more formal reviews, in this case after four
weeks. Here again, however, the emphasis was not so much on how well the
client was meeting the employer's needs per se as on enabling the client to
address any problems and develop into the job. To this end, the reviews them-

selves were very different from those at Project A, in that a structured process was used to enable the client and their manager to provide feedback to each other. Before each review, both the client and manager were asked to complete an assessment form. These forms were returned to the project worker before the review and were then used as the starting point for discussion. Once each party had provided feedback to the other, the worker would summarise what had been said and, where it seemed necessary, encourage the client and manager to set goals for extending the client's skills and experience. As one client remembered this:

> I think [the project worker] pushed for me a bit... when she knew I was ready to move on, instead of doing basic things. She used to say, well what else is there [the client] can do? And then my supervisor off the floor used to be brought in and they'll say, well we'll give her a trial on collect by car.

At the end of each review, the question of whether further reviews were needed was raised and a date agreed for the next review if required. Thus both the frequency of subsequent reviews and the length of time over which the worker would remain involved were a matter for ongoing negotiation.

## The underpinning models of recovery

In essence, the two approaches to employment support described above were underpinned by contrasting models of the nature of recovery from mental health problems. At Project A, the approach was clearly underpinned by a clinical model within which clients referred to the project were seen as needing to move from being ill to being more or less well again before getting a job. From this perspective, the primary purpose of employment support was one of enabling clients at the 'convalescent' stage, that is those who were not yet sufficiently well, to become ready for work. Once clients were perceived to be ready for work, they were treated as autonomous, independent adults who could be expected to fit into and function in the workplace like anyone else.

At Project D, clients were not expected to have put their problems behind them before starting work. From the perspective of workers at this project, clients' mental health problems were seen as having ongoing potential implications for work and they were not expected to be able to quickly fit into and function in a job unaided. Rather, the approach was based on an assumption of interdependency and initial vulnerability. In turn, clients' recovery and entry to work were seen in terms of an ongoing, incremental process involving adaptation and adjustment in the interaction between the individual and the work environment, a process in which they would inevitably require support, at least for some time.

This second model has considerable resonance with the rethinking of recovery that is gaining ground in the field of mental health, particularly in relation to seeing work as a significant stage in the journey to recovery, rather than recovery as a necessary precursor to work.[1]

## Strengths and limitations

It should be stressed that this research was not designed as an evaluative study and we are not therefore able to draw firm conclusions about the comparative effectiveness of the two approaches we have described. However, the accounts of clients, project workers and managers did highlight some strengths and limitations, which in certain circumstances appeared to have a bearing on clients' ability to retain their job. In weighing up these strengths and limitations, we focus in turn on the two models of recovery underpinning the two approaches.

### The clinical recovery model

From one perspective, a strength of the approach underpinned by a clinical understanding of recovery was the speed with which some clients were able to move into paid work. As Justine Schneider shows in Chapter 5, previous research in the United States indicates that rapid job finding with minimal prevocational job preparation is more effective in enabling clients to find and retain jobs than approaches that emphasise the need for longer job preparation. However, the success of this approach in the United States also depends on features lacking within the approach at Project A, including attention to clients' individual preferences, continuous assessment and ongoing support.

In the two cases from Project A where clients were able to retain their jobs, a lengthier process of assessment and preparation was arguably unnecessary but in the other two cases there were indications that the process was insufficiently thorough. In one case, the client explained that his expectations of employment support had included assistance not only with preparing for and finding a job but also with understanding the implications for employment of his mental health problems. However, this help had not been forthcoming and the client experienced a recurrence of his mental health problems within a matter of weeks. The second client also began to experience problems soon after starting work and she too lost her job. In this case the client had been encouraged to return to her previous job with an agency providing care for older people, with little assessment of her needs. Her account suggests that a more detailed assessment would have indicated alternative career options.

> I didn't feel I wanted to do that any more. I don't know, I felt like I had elderly people all my life and I always looked after my grandmother and for my sick mother... I didn't want to do elderly care because I found this very stressful and if you are a sufferer from depression it's not necessarily helpful... I was desperate for permanent work... I wanted something permanent with a regular income.

A further limitation of the clinical model of recovery stemmed from the view of clients assessed as ready to look for work as independent, autonomous adults who required no further help. The accounts of clients from Project A suggest that when they were left to raise their needs themselves, they were unlikely to do so. In one case where the client lost his job within weeks, for example, moving from an unpaid placement to paid work had meant an early start with a long journey to work, as well as taking on full-time hours. This client experienced particular difficulty in the mornings, a not uncommon problem as Mo Hutchison's account in Chapter 3 demonstrates, and his energy levels were also low, due to the side effects of his medication. However, he did not raise the implications of this with his manager when he was offered paid work. As he commented with hindsight:

> I think I may have taken on too much, I remember the shift was an early shift and I found that hard. . . I used to get up at a quarter to six, five-thirty to get there for seven. . . I think it was maybe I wasn't getting enough sleep or something. . . I don't know, it was just generally I would get a bit hyperactive and not talking very coherently, there were various symptoms that go with it.

Another client had been able to retain her job but had encountered problems that had driven her to the brink of resignation. Although she did eventually contact the project and received advice that she greatly appreciated, she had been discouraged from making contact until the problem had reached crisis point.

> Well I think when I got the job I thought that was it. . . To tell you the truth I phoned up in desperation. I didn't feel I could phone . . . They've got people to find jobs for. . . I try not to bother them.

## The social recovery model

In many ways, working within a social recovery model avoided the limitations of the clinical model. As has been seen, the job-finding process at Project D was based on a detailed assessment of clients' skills and needs coupled with careful consideration of the extent to which a job would match these. Equally, follow-up support was negotiated with both clients and managers as a matter of course and there appears to have been no question at Project D of clients moving into work without support. An initial indication of the strength of this approach was that all three clients from the project had been able to retain their jobs for a considerable period of time. However, before jumping to conclusions it is necessary to consider whether the intensity of the approach might be unwelcome to some clients and to some workplace managers.

Taking the assessment and job preparation process first, none of the clients from Project D had found the assessment and preparation process intrusive. Rather, this appears to have been a key factor in developing the confidence to make their way into work. A feature that appeared to offset the risk that the assessment and job preparation process would be seen as intrusive was the clear employment-related rationale for exploring mental health and personal issues. On the other hand, as has been seen, one of the clients from Project A would have welcomed more help with these issues. However, the length of the process at Project D was a potentially greater limitation. In the light of the North American evidence, greater flexibility in relation to the length of assessment would arguably strengthen the approach.

Turning to job finding and follow-up support, it is again arguable that some clients and managers might find the approach taken at Project D overly intrusive.

From the clients' perspective, the primary reason clients from Project A gave for not taking up the support that was available during job club hours was their concern to be able to cope independently. For these clients, then, the approach taken at Project D might have been seen as overprotective. However, there was some evidence that the way in which support was offered at Project A may have contributed to clients' reluctance to use it. As one of the interview extracts cited earlier indicates, the restricted hours for contact coupled with the project's emphasis on autonomy and independence appears to have left clients with the message that they shouldn't 'bother' the project workers by seeking support.

In contrast, at Project D clients' perception of the support available through the formal review process was not couched in terms of dependency but in terms of a process designed to enable them to grow into their job. Far from being perceived as overprotective, the way in which ongoing support was offered was perceived as a boost to clients' confidence which enabled them to make their own way independently. As this client put it:

> She just said if there was any problems whatsoever give her a ring and we would sort them out. But she said, I don't think you'll need me. She gives people confidence in that way. She knows how far people can push themselves I think... It's like carrying a tablet around and you're never going to get a headache.

On the basis of the available evidence, it therefore appears that the approach of leaving clients to initiate follow-up support carried a risk that they would interpret using support in terms of dependency. Somewhat paradoxically, when the provision of follow-up support was not optional, clients did not view this as intrusive or overprotective, perhaps because it was standard practice and to that extent not a matter of their personal independence. On these grounds, the advantages of an incremental and ongoing understanding of 'recovery' in relation to job finding and follow-up support appear to have outweighed any disadvantages from the clients' perspective.

Where workplace managers' views were concerned, the impression from some of those involved with clients from Project A was that they did not expect more support than they received, raising the question of whether these managers would have found the approach at Project D intrusive. However, this manager at least would clearly have welcomed more support than she received.

> I think the big concern is once their work placement is successful and we decide to offer them a position... it's how we deal with any future problems... The individual has to request that [the project] step back in if there is a problem... So that can be quite difficult. Because if [the project] don't know there is a problem, then they're not able to offer support and we can't go to them and say because that's an infringement on that person.

The length of time for which the clients interviewed from Project D had held their jobs meant only one manager who had been closely involved with the project was still in post at the time of the research interviews. From this manager's perspective the provision of support had been welcome.

Her role was very much a facilitator. I think if there had been problems I could have gone back to her at any point. She was always going to be there, checking on how he was doing, from his point of view and ours, and she was there if there were any problems and we could go straight to her if need be and she would pick them up directly, if there was anything I couldn't address with him.

In another case, the project worker's own account suggests that the approach must have been appreciated, in that the company concerned had adopted the project's formal review process for their own appraisal procedures.

On balance, then, it appears that the strengths of the social recovery model again outweighed any limitations in terms of the implications for managers.

## Discussion

Although our sample was small, the data obtained clearly highlight the advantages of an approach to employment support underpinned by an understanding of recovery as an ongoing social process. While we did not set out to evaluate the effectiveness of these two approaches, our results do suggest that this approach offers a more promising way forward for supported employment in the UK. This argument is strengthened by the close approximation of the approach at Project D, with the exception of the length of assessment, to the Individual Placement and Support (IPS) approach supported by evaluation studies (*see* Chapter 5).

As noted earlier, the salience of the notion of recovery as an ongoing experience or journey is gaining ground in the field of mental health. However, our study highlights two potential problems in implementing approaches grounded in this model in the context of employment support as currently practised at the projects we studied.

First, the range of expertise required of employment support workers in working within a social recovery model was striking. Not only must workers be comfortable with exploring mental health and other personal issues with clients. They must also be familiar with the world of work and able both to work with clients on work-related issues and to negotiate effectively with employers. As Justine Schneider points out in the previous chapters, the integration of vocational expertise within community mental health teams is a key aspect of the IPS approach. In the cases we studied, however, even liaison between the employment support projects and mental health services was minimal. It seems reasonable to suggest that the ready access to support from mental health professionals provided by integration would both reduce the length of the assessment process and address the issue of the extent of expertise required of employment project workers.

Second, integration could enhance the capacity to assist clients who experience mental health problems while at work to keep their job and, importantly, to enable them to gain the ability to manage their problems themselves. Neither Project A nor Project D appeared to engage in this kind of work with clients. However, this is an issue that professionals with skills in cognitive therapy would be well placed to address, as this extract from an interview with a client at a third employment project illustrates.

> One of the things that I could have shown you today was a sort of analysis that [my community psychiatric nurse] did of my relapse. Where basically I had delusions of self-importance, and communication with the family and communication with work breaks down. And it's realising those symptoms and being able to tackle them before it's too late really.

## Conclusion

Our study augments Justine Schneider's overview of approaches to employment support in the previous chapter by exploring variations in approach in greater depth. The results highlight the strengths of adopting a social recovery model in providing employment support. They also highlight the importance of working towards the integration of vocational expertise within community mental health teams. This would address the wide-ranging role demands placed on employment support workers. Crucially, integration could also facilitate timely, comprehensive assessment, support clients in managing their mental health and prevent job loss through swift intervention when clients in work experience mental ill health.

## Reference

1 Ridgway P (2001) ReStorying psychiatric disability: learning from first person recovery narratives. *Psychiatric Rehabilitation Journal.* **24**(4): 335–43.

# Chapter 8

# Putting the community back into community care

Patience Seebohm

## Introduction

People employed within community mental health services have chosen a career that is immensely challenging and potentially rewarding and enriching. Their work to support people in moving from crisis and despair towards a renewed sense of strength, independence and well-being should be creative and fulfilling.

Yet research suggests these ambitions may be pursued at a personal cost and with unsatisfactory results. Community mental health professionals, particularly social workers and community psychiatric nurses (CPNs), often experience low morale, emotional exhaustion and 'burnout'.[1] Where morale is low, outcomes for people using services may be adversely affected.[2] Few people attending community teams take up paid employment[3] or get help to tackle the discrimination and stigma which may have a more damaging and long-term disabling impact than their ill health. In fact, many people who use mental health services feel the services are themselves discriminatory, failing to listen to or respect their aspirations.[4] It is argued that people get little help to be 'socially included' within their neighbourhood despite receiving community-based services.[5]

Instead of helping people to get out of their rooms and into college or voluntary and paid work, instead of helping them to use local leisure facilities and make new friends, community team staff report a preoccupation with risk assessment.[2] Staff may not want to work in this way but they face many pressures which combine to cause a focus on personal and public safety. They may have limited encouragement or time to help people move out of their 'comfort zone' and take the risk of a new and interesting but daunting venture in the local community. High caseloads may be partly – but by no means entirely – responsible for reinforcing this risk-averse approach, which is determined by the *use* as well as the *amount* of time available.

The good news is that there are increasing numbers of people at all levels of mental health services who are changing the focus of their work. They are breaking down the physical and psychological separation of the community team from the variety, potential and wealth of their local area. Many are driving forward a new vision of their purpose, by seeking ways of validating the 'community' aspect to mental health services, building partnerships, changing attitudes, gaining new skills and more flexible ways of working. This chapter draws on our study of three NHS trusts[6] that are seeking these kinds of changes in relation to employment, on our experience of supporting those attempting to find new ways of working and on the work of other writers and researchers, to look at some of the concerns and achievements of community-based mental health staff, their service users and senior managers. Evidence from our study and from other research suggests that a new way of working may not reduce staff workload but can make a powerful and beneficial impact on both service users and their professional support staff, as they find a renewed sense of purpose and achievement. In the following sections we describe the three sites that took part in our study and discuss their experiences in relation to six issues:

- the challenge of developing a new vision
- introducing and working with vocational expertise
- communication, respect and trust
- influence and guidance
- tapping into community resources
- finding allies in black and minority ethnic community groups.

## The study sites

The three study sites, described here as sites A, B and C, were chosen to facilitate exploration of different approaches to increasing service users' access to vocational expertise. Site A had recently completed a 12-month pilot project involving the appointment of a vocational specialist to work with two community mental health teams (CMHTs), in line with the Individual Placement and Support (IPS) approach. Site B had a vocational specialist based within an industrial therapy unit. His responsibilities included providing a vocational support service to all community team and day service clients. Site C had developed a model of vocational support that involved allocating a vocational lead role to an occupational therapist (OT) within each CMHT. The OTs were supported and advised by a vocational specialist responsible for the whole locality and employed by the trust.

Since the aim was to explore participants' experiences, qualitative data collection methods were used. These comprised semi-structured interviews with team staff who held care coordinator responsibilities, the vocational specialists and other professionals identified by local staff as important resources in providing employment support to clients.

## The challenge of developing a new vision

Our study found that in all three sites some managers, staff and service users were calling for community mental health services to instil hope in those who use their services and to take their need for a decent home, friends and a valued occupation at least as seriously as diagnosis and medication. This is now becoming a familiar theme in mental health[7] reinforced by the recent Social Exclusion Unit report.[8] However, even where there is commitment at a senior level, changes in focus and ways of working are hard to implement. Many professionals have been trained in and grown accustomed to a more medical approach and their attitudes may be hard to shift. Consequently, the new rhetoric some-times turns out to be just another way of doing things within the same institutional framework.

For instance, some trusts are looking to 'social firms' to provide work oppor-tunities for their service users. Businesses accurately described as social firms can make a useful contribution where they are part of a spectrum of employ-ment opportunities. However, the term is sometimes used to describe work activities identified as the safe and therefore preferred option for people using day services and these then start to look like a new form of sheltered employ-ment.[9] Similarly, voluntary work can be an important element in a spectrum of opportunities but if voluntary work placements are developed within the mental health trust for an indefinite period with no planned or supported route into paid employment, this confines mental health service users to unemploy-ment and potential exploitation. Even paid employment for a few service users within a trust may be progress but does not indicate a fundamental change of vision or direction, unless accompanied by new support systems and major changes in the practices of occupational health and human resources depart-ments, and team managers.

> A lot of the good work that's happened here has been very insular and doesn't fit into the wider community, if anything, it's quite insti-tutional, it's a new type of institutional thinking... it's not actually about people having roles in the community you know, or having jobs out there in the wide world. (Senior manager, site B)

A further force for resistance to the new agenda is the UK government's focus on public protection, fuelled by a small number of tragic incidents that have generated adverse publicity. This adds to the complexity of the challenge facing mental health services but should not lead to oppressive services for the vast majority of people with mental health problems. Risk assessments can be used to determine what a person *can* do and what risks they *can* take, just as power-fully as indicating what risks should be avoided. The need to avoid risk can be used to argue for improved, integrated support services, to ensure that people can access the help they need as they move forward in their lives. Failure to provide this integrated approach can result in people either not moving forward at all or taking on a job without easy access to help when they need it. As Jenny Secker and colleagues illustrate in Chapter 7, the consequence may be job loss and ill health, through no fault of individual support staff but through a failure to work together on employment issues.

Despite concern for public protection, the call for mainstream mental health services to actively support social inclusion remains loud and clear. The govern-ment recognises the reduced risk of self-harm for those in employment and requires mental health services to take this into account when shaping their services.[10] There is also a range of policy documents promoting social inclu-sion.[8,11] Citizenship is becoming a familiar word in a mental health context. Civil rights are being asserted: the right to work, to respect, to choice and to freedom from discrimination.[12] It is argued that the mental health world needs to move on into a 'new phase of development'.[13]

## Introducing and working with vocational expertise

A key element of the new vision is enabling people to obtain paid employment in ordinary jobs. This requires introducing vocational expertise, both from specialist staff but also to some extent within the core skills of CPNs, social workers, psychologists and psychiatrists. They all have an important role to play in helping their service users achieve sustainable, rewarding and enjoyable employment (as we all hope to achieve). Financial investment by the NHS (new or reallocated) is required to bring in the vocational expert but it costs nothing to set a clear mandate for all mental health staff to jointly contribute to employment support.

In our study of three sites, we found community mental health staff varied in their response to the notion of sharing the task of providing vocational support. A small number of staff (of all disciplines) entered wholeheartedly into this, seeing it as central to their role but some passed over all responsibility to the 'vocational expert' and did not perceive vocational issues to be relevant to their own job. Others felt that they themselves had the necessary expertise, although there was little evidence to support this view. At site C, where the teams participating in the study had allocated a specialist vocational role to their occupational therapists, the care coordinators and key workers played little part in vocational support, despite the rhetoric of partnership working. At site B, the vocational specialist was located in a different building. Although the clinicians expressed a wish to work with him for the benefit of service users, the vocational expert did not appreciate the value of a joint approach, taking a stance similar to the clinical recovery model described in the previous chapter.

> We're more interested in the person's future so we don't phone the key worker for any sort of assessment or past medical history or anything like that. (Vocational specialist, site B)

Unfortunately, staff and vocational specialists who felt no need to work together effectively denied service users access to specialist information and support. At site A, on the other hand, the IPS philosophy was embedded in the attitude and practice of the vocational expert and senior management and was supported by the psychiatrist and it was at this site that working relations between clinicians and vocational experts were found to be closest. Even clinicians who were initially sceptical came to believe in the value of joint working as the service developed. Not only did it improve the lives of their service users but it also lightened the pressure upon the staff themselves who gained satisfaction from improved outcomes.

As a result, at site A the staff felt able to help any person who was motivated to try for an ordinary job in the locality. No one who wanted to get an ordinary job was excluded and this gave satisfaction to both staff and service users.

> She's one of the most difficult people we have on our whole caseload in the team and to find something... was quite difficult... it took a lot of time, a lot of effort, and a lot of work... but it was worth it. (CPN, site A)

## Communication, respect and trust

The primary factor in developing good interprofessional working identified in our study was the shared vision of an integrated service. At site A, just such a vision provided a clear lead right through from the chief executive, senior managers and psychiatrists to the team leaders, influencing how staff understood their role and spent their time.

> She [the team manager] was a CPN... just had a passionate belief about people in the service having opportunities...I think knowing that was valued by her was a good influence on the team. (OT, site A)

This commitment to a positive, integrated approach to vocational issues has to be shared by the vocational expert. Instead of taking the independent approach described above, the vocational worker will only win respect and cooperation if he or she, in turn, respects and values the contribution of clinical staff.

> You can't do the vocational without the clinical... I have a respect for the clinician's expertise and their background knowledge of the client... the key worker's crucial. (Vocational specialist, site A)

Our research concluded that this consistent lead and vision, backed up by structural change and new financial priorities, is essential if we want to guarantee a different experience for service users. Implementing the vision, once the structural and financial changes are made, requires easy, frequent, formal and informal communication.

> It's constant communication and collaboration, with the client, key worker, myself all in agreement. (Vocational specialist, site A)

Communication helps to build the trust necessary for good collaboration. Mental health professionals will not want to refer their service users to others unless assured of their competence. Vocational activity can improve health and may engage those who are still experiencing symptoms of ill health and lacking in self-esteem. Their professional support staff will want to be assured that, if they make a referral to the vocational expert, the outcome is not likely to be harmful. In our three-site study, the necessary trust was established through frequent and easy communication with some staff quite quickly but with others, it took a period of time. Staff stability was therefore an important factor in success.

Location and office design were found to make a significant difference to easy communications. Much learning and trust grew during informal conversations over coffee, where staff of different disciplines, including the vocational expert, met for problem solving and sharing experiences. Team stability and investment in professional development enabled trusting relationships to become established. Where vocational expertise is lodged within an external agency or is geographically separate, this level of communication, respect and trust will be much harder, if not impossible, to establish.

Formal communications were also important, including invitations to Care Programme Approach (CPA) and other case reviews. An invitation to attend reviews acknowledges the contribution of the vocational expert and makes it possible to tap their knowledge of the service user when making important decisions about their future. Similarly, if clinical staff visit employment projects, this can help to increase trust in their work and raise expectations for their service users.

Stories of successful service users who have been supported by NHS colleagues make an impact, whether this communication is over coffee, in the trust newsletter or by presentations from the service users themselves. Staff will be interested to hear of the benefits not only to the service users but also to their professional colleagues, who may have been able to reduce the level of support as the service user regained confidence.

Data collected on the numbers of service users entering employment, education and voluntary work can, if analysed and reported back to individual teams, help staff to compare their ways of working and sends a positive message back to those who are doing well.

Staff with academic interests and psychiatrists in particular may come to value new ways of working by seeing research data on the benefits of employment and the harmful effects of unemployment. For others, communication with a range of workers with whom they work in partnership (employment, housing, leisure staff) can help to broaden understanding of 'what works' for mental health service users. The limitations of the medical model will become apparent as other ways of helping people to regain their well-being are understood.

## Influence and guidance

Our study also found that clear guidance to clinical staff helped them to demystify vocational issues, which are unlikely to be covered during their professional training, leaving clinicians feeling disempowered and uncomfortable in this area of work. Torrey has provided practical information illustrating the kind of help clinical, social work and support staff can provide.[14]

- Helping service users and clinical teams have realistic vocational expectations.
- Coordinating service users' clinical and rehabilitation plans and interventions.
- Providing basic support and problem solving to service users.
- Contributing their insight to appropriate job matches that will support service users' health management as well as vocational needs.
- Helping service users manage their mental health problems.
- Helping families adjust to the service user's employment.
- Helping support service users' long-term rehabilitation efforts by keeping a positive frame of mind.

The overriding message from Torrey and others is that vocational support should not be seen as an additional task for clinical staff who already feel overburdened but as requiring simply a shift in the kinds of questions clinicians ask.

Perhaps the most important contribution that clinicians can offer (and the contribution often most valued) is positive encouragement, a 'can do' attitude that spreads self-confidence and a determination to succeed. As Bob Grove and Helen Membrey demonstrate in Chapter 1, motivation to get a job is a key factor in success for service users moving into work and clinical staff play a crucial role in developing this.

> They [clinicians] have this very positive influence, so very very crucial. (Vocational specialist, site A)

Case supervision and reviews can be used to remind clinical staff that work is achievable if the individual wants it. If the first steps into employment are not successful, then clinical staff and their service users can be reassured that setbacks are normal for all of us and do not imply that it was a mistake to try. The attitude of team managers and psychiatrists, backed up by trust policy and chief executives, is crucial to support staff in opening up opportunities where earlier they might have only seen risk.

> Dr A is actually the one who most values work, he will suggest work in places where I wouldn't have... that's good to discuss it and look at the potential. (Social worker, site A)

Caseloads must be at a manageable level and it has been suggested that 25 is the maximum where positive and creative support can take place.[15] Managers can encourage flexible working hours, with support meetings taking place near the workplace or college so that people can take up full-time employment *and* maintain their support, which they may perceive to be a lifeline.

Staff can be advised to keep open the files of people who begin to attend an employment support service, instead of closing the case soon after referral. The first weeks of transition into employment may involve intense work but in the long term, dependency on mental health services is likely to be reduced. However, as noted above, quick access to mental health support can be a crucial factor in job retention.

Staff training on vocational issues is likely to appear most inspirational and less threatening if it is delivered firstly by people who have used services, and who can describe the help they received, and secondly by colleagues of the same profession who champion employment support as central to their professional role. Each profession has a particular contribution to make. This might include finding the right medication to suit a person's lifestyle, working with their family, helping them to function effectively in the workplace or developing their social skills. The new way of working can be introduced as a way of enhancing professional skills and confidence.

A manager who appears to be making yet another demand on staff will not be welcomed. In view of the immense pressures of workload and responsibilities facing mental health professionals, it may be useful to emphasise the ways in which these can be managed more easily through sharing the burden and enjoying increased rewards.

Influence from colleagues can be more subtle than guidance or training and at least as powerful. In particular, colleagues who have used mental health services bring a new perspective and give a new, positive image of what can be achieved. Increasing numbers of mental health trusts are recruiting people who have used mental health services to specified 'user' posts, with a mix of success as some professionals have initially found it difficult to trust and respect a former 'patient' as colleague.[16] People who have used services often have a deep commitment to helping others who come after them[17] but many have argued that it is best if specified user posts are replaced with an opportunity to compete on an equal basis with others for any job within the trust, with their particular expertise valued in the recruitment process. Disclosure of their health will then be a personal matter, as it would be for any other member of staff, and they have equal rights in this respect. Their values and experience will still influence other staff, perhaps in subtler, quieter ways.

An example of this is to be found on a ward in Sheffield, where one member of staff, also a service user, got permission to run weekly advice sessions on employment on his ward. Although his post was ward based, he got permission to take people out to sort out employment and training before discharge, to make hospital admission less harmful.[18]

The vision, communication, guidance and influence described above can give clinical staff all they need to work with their vocational experts and support their service users to achieve their ambitions. Their work becomes less focused on prevention of harm and more on the realisation of individual aspirations and is therefore immediately more creative and exciting.

## Tapping into community resources

People who use community mental health services will need more than the expertise of their care coordinator and vocational worker to recover a rounded, fulfilling life. Community agencies and local people have a lot to offer but ill health and the discrimination that follows may leave people with mental health problems isolated and reluctant to make contact. Community mental health services, including both clinical staff and vocational experts, can tap into these local resources and help to break down the barriers.[19]

> The incorporation of evidence-based practice within vocational rehabilitation into the clinical teams has led to a shift from a purely medical outcome to a social outcome... the teams are now more socially connected with their communities.

An essential partner will be a source of benefits advice 'on tap' when people are moving into work, training or study. Our study in three sites found welfare rights advice problematic at all three and the widespread ignorance of clinicians about benefits issues was of particular concern. Some staff had an unfounded confidence in their own expertise. This created additional barriers to work and may have meant that individuals did not receive their full in-work entitlements. A partnership with an independent agency to provide immediate, expert advice may need to be supported by funding, due to the operational pressure experienced by most independent welfare rights agencies. The advantages of investing in this for the trust will be the increased confidence and pace at which service users will move into vocational activities.

In addition to arrangements with an independent service, community mental health services can receive invaluable help from JobCentre Plus for their service users' welfare benefits and job search. The vocational expert serving the community mental health team will work very closely with JobCentre Plus but it is important that clinical staff also feel comfortable dealing with Jobcentre personal advisors, disability employment advisors and other staff to help support their service users into work. JobCentre Plus is trying to address the lack of trust and understanding between its advisors and people with mental health problems, partly through outreach services, and it may be possible to establish an outreach service at a comfortable location, maybe within a day service.

The neighbourhood and wider locality will have a wide range of employers, community groups, self-help groups, spiritual and religious centres and others that all have something to offer.[20]

> The reality is that community groups can and do want to help but we as professionals don't go and ask them...These are groups which see people in the streets acting strange, having arguments outside the bus stop, people who are unwell. They're not going to change their ideas unless we go and tell them we have a wealth of talent.

Many employment workers make the same point: ask employers and others to accept mental health service users within their organisation and often there is a positive response. As the study described in Chapter 7 illustrates, the discriminatory attitudes of employers can dissipate when someone speaks with authority and confidence about a job applicant's suitability for a vacant post and offers support when needed.

This can open up opportunities for a wide range of interesting work experience, leisure and social activities. People who have been unwell may be seeking a change of direction; young people may be uncertain of what their skills and aspirations are and may be motivated to try out new activities. The range of organisations which can offer these kinds of opportunities is enormous, from steam engine preservation groups to nature conservation organisations or the local CD shop and dance club.[21] It will help if mental health staff can work confidently with these, as and when necessary, although the lead role in developing partnerships may be taken by a vocational expert or non-clinical member of staff.

Home tutoring and specialist provision at college may be available in the local area or could be developed with support from community mental health services. The emphasis needs to be on enabling people to move on to mainstream provision at the earliest opportunity. Confidence increases as skills return and increase and the expense of such a service may be recouped through reduced medication, support and entry to employment.

Professionals may anticipate and fear rejection from people outside the field, reflecting their own assumption that service users are more likely to experience long-term disability than reveal a wealth of talent. Yet if these professionals instead had confidence in their service users' potential, they could instil confidence in others who may have no information apart from often negative media coverage.

As people with mental health problems start to take up training and work, it is appropriate that they should begin to tap into alternative sources of support. The neighbourhood may be rich in opportunities for this, in the workplace or at college, with local community groups, interest groups, churches and other spiritual centres. Access to natural supports such as these can be fostered or facilitated alongside clinical support, so that in time friendships may develop and reduce the need for professional help.

## Finding allies in black and minority ethnic community groups

Community agencies led by and serving people from black and minority ethnic groups can have immense value, if they have an acceptance and understanding of mental health issues. Once again, joint working is more helpful to the service user than a referral and case closure but the role of the mental health professional will need to be explored with the individual and his or her community agency.

It is well documented that statutory services have difficulty addressing the mental health needs of black and minority ethnic groups.[22] Fear, on the part of both professionals and service users alike, plays a part in this[23] but institutional and direct racism is found within the NHS as it is within our other institutions, exacerbating the problem of low expectations for people with a mental health diagnosis.

Specialist employment services for people with mental health problems often fail to attract proportionate numbers of black and Asian service users,[24, 25] but anecdotal evidence suggests that employment support is highly valued if it is offered in a format which is accessible and acceptable. As one staff member at a black voluntary organisation put it:

> He has been working on his CV. He wants to go into bus driving... I spoke to his social worker and he said 'It's unbelievable...No one has ever been able to engage with him'.

Integrated vocational and mental health support can be achieved and acceptable for this population. Key factors in success suggested by preliminary investigations indicate the importance of a location in the community, flexible ways of working, an encouraging, can-do attitude and partners who can offer expertise and opportunities free from discrimination. Peer support helps to restore hope which may have been crushed by education, health and employment services.[26] As a result of their experiences, some black service users may lack the self-esteem or social skills needed to cope with the multiple pressures of racism and mental health stigma.[23] Black-led services can help to restore a positive sense of identity and help people to develop ways of coping with day-to-day experiences in the workplace.

Employment services based within black and minority ethnic agencies fulfil a useful function but, as with community teams, they need stability to establish effective partnerships and this requires secure funding. Moreover, potential partners such as colleges, JobCentre Plus and welfare rights agencies may themselves need training or resources before they have the language, skills or confidence to provide a service easily accessed by black clients. Funding arrangements can prove difficult as many black and minority ethnic agencies aim to support those in need (regardless of diagnosis) and to provide services not usually included in care planning. To achieve joint working with these agencies, mental health professionals, senior managers and commissioners need to look beyond the medical model of mental distress and open their minds to new ways of doing things.

At all levels within the NHS, there are psychiatrists and staff exploring ways of working that are more responsive to the needs of black and minority ethnic communities[27] but they remain at this time a minority force. However, there are mental health professionals, maybe many, who are aware of the need to improve provision for their black service users and who, given the opportunity, would welcome partners who can support them in this.

## Conclusion

The fundamental shift required by mental health professionals is to find new ways of working with new colleagues and partners. This can appear daunting, even alarming, unless management and staff can agree on a clear and achievable goal. A defined purpose avoids the pressure of apparently incompatible demands which can burden mental health professionals.

Many service users are asking for services not to aim at stability, safety or maintenance at the expense of stimulation and personal fulfilment. The goal now sought by many people is 'recovery', not in the clinical sense with an endpoint of stability but in the social sense of finding a new way of living a fulfilled life in the community, managing their health problems and gaining sufficient control over their lives to enjoy the security of a decent home, a good job, a circle of friends and the opportunity to exercise civil rights.

If people want to live without a high intake of drugs which leaves them lethargic and their life grey, there may be no guarantee of freedom from symptoms of ill health. However, occasional periods of ill health become less damaging if services help people to maintain their job, home and social networks during these difficult times and enable them to return to normal activities as quickly as possible.

Once clinical staff are reassured that they will not be blamed for every hospital admission, they can enjoy encouraging their service users to try out new ventures and then share enjoyment of the increased confidence and well-being that are likely to follow. The workload may be the same but the rewards will be much greater. Staff working in this way, with a range of partners and connections in the local community, have a great 'toolbox' of resources, as well as a team which can share pressures, problem solving and setbacks.

The message from our study of the three sites taking on the challenges we have described is that where vocational and mental health support are integrated, the work can be both exhilarating and supportive.

You're not just an isolated person, you're suddenly a force... I personally felt more empowered by that, and the more empowered I feel that has a knock-on effect for the clients. (Vocational specialist, site A)

# References

1 Prosser D, Johnson S, Kuipers E *et al.* (1999) Mental health, burnout and job satisfaction in a longitudinal study of mental health staff. *Social Psychiatry and Psychiatric Epidemiology.* **34**: 295–300.

2 Priebe S, Fakhoury W, Hoffman K *et al.* (2005) Morale and job perception of community mental health professionals in Berlin and London. *Social Psychiatry and Psychiatric Epidemiology.* **40**(3): 223–32.

3 Perkins R and Rinaldi M (2002) A decade of rising employment. *Psychiatric Bulletin.* **26**: 295–8.

4 Sayce L (2002) Beyond good intentions: making anti-discrimination strategies work. *Disability and Society.* **18** (5): 625–42.

5 Barr A, Henderson P and Stenhouse C (2001) *Tackling Social Exclusion Through Social Care Practice.* Joseph Rowntree Foundation, York.

6 Seebohm P and Secker J (2003) Increasing the vocational focus of the community mental health team. *Journal of Interprofessional Care.* **17**(3): 281–91.

7 Repper J and Perkins R (2003) *Social Inclusion and Recovery.* Bailliere Tindall, London.

8 OPDM (2004) *Mental Health and Social Exclusion. Social Exclusion Unit Report.* Office of the Deputy Prime Minister, London.

9 Secker J, Dass S and Grove B (2003) The organisation and operation of social firms. *Disability and Society.* **18**(5): 659–74.

10 Department of Health (2004) *Health and Social Care Planning Framework and Targets for 2005–2008.* Department of Health, London.

11 NIMHE (2004) *From Here to Equality.* National Institute for Mental Health England, Leeds.

12 Wallcraft J with Read J and Sweeney A (2003) *On Our Own Terms.* Sainsbury Centre for Mental Health, London.

13 Sayce L (2000) *From Psychiatric Patient to Citizen.* Mind, London.

14 Torrey W (1998) Practice guidelines for clinicians working in programmes providing integrated vocational and clinical services for persons with severe mental disorders. *Psychiatric Rehabilitation Journal.* **21**(4): 388–93.

15 Becker D and Drake R (2003) *A Working Life for People with Severe Mental Illness.* Oxford University Press, Oxford.

16 Gell C and Seebohm P (2001) *Valuing Experience.* Institute for Applied Health and Social Policy, King's College London, London.

17 Ridgway P (2001) ReStorying psychiatric disability: learning from first person recovery narratives. *Psychiatric Rehabilitation Journal.* **22**(4): 335–43.

18 Seebohm P and Gell C (2003) *Review of Unlocking Potential Year 2.* Sainsbury Centre for Mental Health, London.

19 Davis M and Rinaldi M (2004) Using an evidence-based approach to enable people with mental health problems to gain and retain employment, education and voluntary work. *British Journal of Occupational Therapy.* **67**(7): 319–22.

20 Seebohm P, Secker J and Grove B (2003) *Hidden Skills, Hidden Talents.* Institute for Applied Health and Social Policy, King's College London, London.

21 Pozner A, Hammond J and Ng M (2000) *Working Together: images of partnership.* Pavilion, Brighton.

22 NIMHE/Department of Health (2003) *Inside Outside: improving mental health services for black and minority ethnic communities in England*. National Institute for Mental Health England, Leeds.

23 Keating F, Robertson D, McCulloch A *et al.* (2002) *Breaking the Circles of Fear: a review of the relationship between mental health services and African and Caribbean communities*. Sainsbury Centre for Mental Health, London.

24 Pozner A, Ng M, Hammond J *et al.* (1996) *Working it Out: creating work opportunities for people with mental health problems*. Pavilion, Brighton.

25 Seebohm P, Cockshutt G, Crawley S *et al.* (2001) *Walsall Mental Health and Employment Research Project*. Institute for Applied Health and Social Policy, King's College London, London.

26 Seebohm P, Jones R and Walker D (2004) *AKABA Baseline Evaluation*. Sainsbury Centre for Mental Health, London.

27 Fernando S (2003) *Cultural Diversity, Mental Health and Psychiatry: the struggle against racism*. Brunner-Routledge, Hove.

# Chapter 9

# A whole-system approach

Rachel Perkins and Miles Rinaldi

## Introduction

Both within and outside the mental health services, diagnoses like schizophrenia and manic depression almost invariably conjure up ideas about deficit and dysfunction, danger and incompetence. The traditional 'deficit-focused' research on which practice within mental health services is founded ensures that workers too often view mental ill health as an entirely negative phenomenon – an irretrievable tragedy for the individual and those around them.[1] The low expectations that too many mental health professionals entertain about those whom they serve are reflected in their bleak prognoses – 'You'll never be able to live independently ... cope with stress ... raise a family ... get a job'.

To be sure, professional negativity may arise from the best of motives: to help people to be 'realistic' about their possibilities, a genuine attempt to protect people from further disappointment, failure and rejection. And notable exceptions to the prevailing wisdom of doom are increasingly to be found among mental health professionals. But it remains the case that the widespread pessimism of too many 'expert' professionals has destructive repercussions for people with mental health problems, the services that they are offered and societal attitudes and beliefs. Nowhere is the vicious cycle of negativity that ensues, more destructive than in the field of employment.

It is very difficult to continue to believe in your own prospects if the experts who are supposed to be helping you tell you that you are too disabled to get a job.[1] But even if you reject the pessimism of the experts, their doom-laden opinions place barriers in your path. If mental health professionals think that employment is an impossible dream then they are unlikely to provide the support and encouragement that may be essential if you are to resume your career or embark on a new one. The numerous 'sheltered workshops' are testimony to the traditional professional opinion that real work is not a realistic possibility, especially for those with more serious and long-standing problems. And of course, employers too often believe the professional experts: if mental health professionals say that people with mental health problems are not capable of working then it is not surprising that employers are reluctant to take you on.

So low professional expectations generate a self-fulfilling prophecy. People with mental health problems and employers alike accede to the opinions of the experts. In the absence of the support and encouragement they need, people give up applying for jobs and employers are reluctant to take them on. The disgracefully high unemployment rates among people with mental health problems that ensue[2] confirm the belief of all – professionals, employers, people with mental health problems themselves and the wider community – that employment is unlikely, if not impossible.

In an attempt to break out of the vicious circle of despair, it is not surprising that those who believe in the possibilities of people with mental health problems have often abandoned mainstream mental health services as a lost cause and sought to establish programmes outside the statutory sector. Such initiatives have doubtless helped many people but they cannot counteract the negative impact of professional advice. If the experts say that work would be too stressful, would exacerbate your problems, then you cease to believe you can work and give up trying to do so. Neither can such initiatives undo the negative impact of powerful professional opinions on employers at both a societal and an individual level, reinforcing the prejudice and discrimination that already exist.

As Patience Seebohm vividly describes in the previous chapter, if a vicious circle of impossibility is to be replaced with a virtuous circle of possibility, a fundamental change of vision and purpose is required throughout mental health services. This may seem a daunting task. It can feel like sitting on the back of an enormous oil tanker on the high seas trying to change its direction by kicking your feet in the water.* But it is possible.

In this chapter we draw upon the experience of almost a quarter of a century of trying to change mental health services and on the lessons learned from 15 years of trying to inculcate the importance of work – the real possibility of employment – into the mainstream work of mental health services in South West London. It has not always been plain sailing, mistakes have been made along the way and there is still a long way to go. But there have been changes.

Until 1990, South West London vocational services comprised a traditional hospital-based industrial therapy unit and a voluntary sector community sheltered workshop established to replace the industrial unit of a long-stay hospital that had closed. Other than prescribing attendance at one of these facilities, work, education and training were rarely considered. By 2004, vocational issues enjoyed a more central place in the work of mental health teams and almost 70% of enhanced care plans contained actions relating to employment, education or other occupation.[3] Twenty employment specialist posts have been created to:

- provide 'individual placement with support'[4–8] to help clients of community mental health, early intervention and assertive outreach teams to access open employment, mainstream voluntary work and education[9]
- provide support to people with mental health problems to get and keep ordinary jobs within the mental health trust itself on the same terms and conditions as all other staff[10–13]
- establish a brief work preparation programme funded by JobCentre Plus.

Together these services annually provide over 1300 people with specialist vocational assistance and each year support in excess of 300 people to get/keep open employment and a further 500 to pursue mainstream education/training, voluntary work, work experience in integrated settings and to access employment services outside the trust (JobCentre Plus, Connexions, specialist voluntary sector employment programmes).

* We are grateful to Geoff Shepherd for introducing us to this analogy.

# The process of change: what have we learnt so far in South West London?

The process of changing the NHS in general, and mental health in particular, has become a veritable industry. The Modernisation Agency, mental health improvement partnerships, regional development centres and numerous practice development networks have spawned innumerable programmes designed to change what services do and how they do it. There have certainly been changes: old asylums have been closed, new teams have been developed, the idea that service users must be involved in the development of services has become firmly entrenched. But equally such initiatives are often less than wholly successful. They fail to win the hearts and minds of staff or to overcome the hurdles of established custom and practice.

Nowhere are these failures more evident than in the field of employment. Research evidence clearly shows that the majority of people with serious mental health problems can gain and sustain employment if they are provided with the right kind of help and support,[5, 7, 8] yet evidence-based support in employment continues to be available to only a tiny proportion of those who could benefit from it. Despite exhortations that employment and education/training form part of enhanced care plans,[3] data are not routinely collected concerning whether this is the case or on exactly how many mental health service users are working.

Our experience in South West London suggests that a number of tactics may be important to raise the profile of work and ensure that vocational issues have a more central place in the work of mental health teams. However, it is important at the outset to emphasise that none of these is more important than the others in changing the way in which systems work – the order in which they are presented here is of no particular significance – and none can stand alone.

## Use outcome and performance measures

With the advent of 'star ratings' and the proliferation of inspections and reviews, measuring the quality and effectiveness of mental health services is a growth industry. This means that performance indicators have become a major driver for service change. And in chasing good ratings, the reality is that the criteria used to evaluate quality and success take on a central importance: if you don't count it, you don't do it.

So we spend time counting the number of new assertive outreach, home treatment and early intervention services, we count how many carer assessments have been carried out, we measure reductions in inpatient bed usage, count care plans ... If vocational issues are to become a central part of services, they have to be part of performance indicators.

Obviously, the national reporting and performance requirements are the most powerful motivators and it is to be hoped that one consequence of the Social Exclusion Unit's report[2] will be to make the measurement of performance in the area of employment/vocational issues a national requirement. However, it is also possible to introduce such indicators as a requirement of local systems.

Commissioners require mental health trusts (and other organisations from whom they contract services) to provide reports of progress against key performance indicators. Negotiations with local commissioners can ensure that indicators relating to employment and vocational issues are included among them. In South West London, for example. the required performance indicators include:

- the proportion of enhanced care plans that include action relating to employment, education/training or other occupation
- the number of people receiving specialist vocational intervention:
  - the number of people supported to get/keep open employment
  - the number of people supported in mainstream education/training and
  - the number of people supported in voluntary work/work experience in open, integrated settings.

Similarly, negotiations with local commissioners and other organisations within the local mental health economy have led to the inclusion of employment outcomes as part of service level agreements with voluntary sector providers. And if you have to count it, it becomes important and you have to do it!

However, a word of caution is warranted. If performance indicators are too extensive and time-consuming to collect, people won't produce the information, so keep it simple and focus on key indicators rather than trying to measure everything. And make sure that the data collected and fed upwards to commissioners are also fed downwards to the professionals who are providing the service and collecting the data so that they too can see the results of their efforts.[14]

## Make use of existing processes

If culture and practice are to be changed, then vocational issues must not only be part of the commissioning agenda, they must also be part of the core business of the organisation as a whole, not just a bolt-on. They must be part of the core organisational processes, such as clinical governance, acute care forums, modernisation and mental health improvement programmes, mental health promotion initiatives, race equality schemes and the agenda of the board.

## Focus on material changes

It is certainly the case that changing philosophies and attitudes is important, but the critical changes that impact on service users are not in the heads of staff but in their behaviour. People need to be clear what behaviours are required and what material changes in outcomes are required if changes are to be effected.

It is often assumed that changes in practice result from changes in principles and attitudes, but causality can operate in the other direction as well: changes in values and philosophy may be a consequence of changes in practice. In South West London initiatives to increase access to employment within mental health services have often been better promoted by working alongside someone who has mental health problems as a colleague than by numerous 'attitude change' initiatives. The imperative 'Just do it!' really can be important in changing hearts and minds.

## Start small and build up

It is clear that, since its inception, the NHS has not been a place where revolutions happen. The process of change is invariably one of progressive reform rather than revolution and the process of real change takes time. Although evidence-based practice is of the essence, the presentation of research findings is not always the best way of changing approaches and practices. At the bottom line, people are more likely to believe that things work if they can see them with their own eyes on their own patch.

If we start small by setting up a pilot in one part of the organisation, then others can see the outcomes with their own eyes and realise that supported employment works not only in Dartmouth, New Hampshire, but also in Tooting, London. It is then easier to roll out the initiatives and increase the pace and scope of changes.

## Capitalise on existing interest, enthusiasm and skills

So which areas should be selected for pilot programmes? There will be pockets of enthusiasm within the organisation and there will also be areas where scepticism is greater. By starting where front-line commitment is greatest – where people are committed to making it work – difficulties can be ironed out before changes are generalised to other areas. Occupational therapists have a key role to play and have been central to the vocational initiatives developed in South West London.

## Ensure assertive, persuasive, credible, senior leadership

Leadership is critical. If widespread organisational changes are to be achieved then leadership must be vested in someone who is sufficiently senior and credible at an organisational level.

Sometimes a separate 'modernisation team' or external consultants are drafted in to facilitate the change process. However, there is a risk that those who are supposed to be spearheading the change will be seen as outsiders who really do not understand the organisation and the issues it faces. If change agents lack credibility and influence within the organisation, their ability to change what happens is limited. Alternatively, responsibility for vocational initiatives may rest in a person or people in one part of the organisation (like the vocational services) that is not really in a position to influence the overall work of the service. Any initiatives developed will be seen as apart from, not a part of, the work of the organisation and their impact on overall philosophy, approach and practice will be limited. To be sure, specialist employment workers and teams are necessary but implanting social inclusion and employment at the heart of the work of services requires that existing influential figures – like chief executives, executive directors, clinical directors, heads of profession, chairs, non-executive directors – play a leading role.

## Start at the top . . .

The idea of 'top-down' change is not always popular but the power of those in high places – for good or ill – should never be underestimated. In the process of developing employment programmes in South West London, there has always been a steady stream of people who go to the chief executive (or the director of nursing or the medical director. . .) and say 'We don't really have to do that, do we?'. It is essential that the answer they get is 'Well, yes, actually, you do'. The active support of key executive directors, the chair and non-executive directors and senior professionals is imperative if organisational change is to be achieved.

## . . . but pay close attention to changing hearts and minds throughout the organisation

Real material change requires active engagement throughout the organisation and most especially the commitment of those front-line managers and senior clinicians who are critical in determining what happens on the ground.

It is important to ensure that dialogue at all levels (from the trust board to meetings with front-line staff) positively encourages people to voice their concerns, however 'politically incorrect' these might be. The 'some people think . . .' approach can be very useful in order to air and address common misconceptions and concerns.

In addition, different people have different beliefs and motivations for working in mental health services and it is necessary to tailor arguments to different audiences: one size does not fit all. In selling the centrality of social inclusion in general, and employment in particular, it is necessary to have a number of cards up your sleeve to appeal to different motivations.

- The research possibilities for aspiring academics.
- The research literature for those who are concerned about delivering evidence-based practice.
- The possibilities for publicity, credit, notoriety for those who want to enhance their own reputation (or that of their service).
- The impact on individual lives and well-being for those whose primary concern is doing something to improve the lives of people with mental health problems.
- The relevance to national targets and priorities for those who must have a weather eye to star ratings.
- Fairness, equity and rights for those whose political concerns predominate.
- Making working life pleasanter, more satisfying, for those who simply want a quiet life.

Also, remember that people hate being taken by surprise. It is grave folly for key managers, commissioners, service users and their representatives, carers groups and so on to hear about proposals second-hand or in a meeting where decisions will be made. They are likely to feel excluded, kept in the dark and their knee-jerk response is likely to be 'no'. Informal chats, telephone conversations, floating ideas at a very early stage and asking others what they think, really enabling people to contribute to the formation of proposals rather than simply commenting when they have been formalised, really crediting a range of people with the development of the ideas, can all be valuable in ensuring eventual acceptance.

## Avoid deskilling existing staff and service users...

Changing the goalposts makes people feel unsafe. Staff may feel deskilled, out of their depth and assume that there is implied criticism of what they have been doing for years, and the natural response is to become defensive and resist change. Service users may feel that support on which they rely is being withdrawn and therefore resist change.

Involvement of service users in the development of new approaches can decrease fears of service change but, as a consequence of professional negativity, many will have lost confidence in their abilities and believe themselves too disabled to work. The change process must include steps to increase confidence and self-belief. However, it is important to involve not only those who use existing services but also those who have been alienated by them. There are as many people – including many from minority ethic communities – who have rejected existing services as irrelevant to their needs and aspirations. Such people can be useful allies in the change process.

On the staff side, the traditional 'guilds' of nursing, occupational therapy, psychiatry, psychology and social work wield an enormous amount of power by defining the scope and standards of their profession, controlling entry to the profession and defining standards of practice, and by vying with each other for supremacy and influence. The power of these professions to impede change should never be underestimated. If vocational issues are to have a central place in mental health services, then each of the guilds must be able to see its unique role in such endeavours. For example, you might argue that:

- nurses provide most of the direct care to clients, therefore their beliefs about the person's capabilities have a critical influence. They will often have a critical role in holding on to hope – believing in people's possibilities when they cannot believe in them themselves. They also have experience of providing the practical help that people need, skills that can be critical in helping someone to work
- occupational therapists have long had a special interest, and central role, in vocational services. Their abilities in the assessment and development of work skills can be central in assisting clients and employers alike to determine what adjustments and supports may be necessary if the person is to work successfully
- psychiatrists have expertise in adjusting medication to maximise functioning and minimise both symptoms and side effects that might impede work performance, and in understanding the functional implications of psychopathology. Their beliefs about a person's capabilities have a great deal of influence over the views of both other staff and employers. If the doctor thinks the person can work, maybe they can
- the therapeutic skills of psychologists (especially cognitive behavioural techniques) can be important not only in decreasing disruptive cognitive and emotional problems but also in helping people to develop ways of managing their symptoms in a work context.

This is not an exhaustive list, merely an illustration of the arguments that might be used to help different professionals to feel less deskilled by changing roles and priorities – to see the critical contribution that they may be able to make to the vocational enterprise.

## ... but ensure the essential specialist skills are there too

While the traditional skills of mental health professionals may be of value in promoting employment opportunities, any change in vision, purpose and goals requires a change in skills. Some of these may be developed as part of the post-qualification training of existing staff and ongoing practice development networks can also be valuable in enabling people to use any new skills and approaches. By working with local training courses, it may be possible to include some of the vocational skills required within pre-qualification training.

However, the specialist expertise required to deliver effective support in employment cannot be seen as a simple 'add-on' to the work and training of existing professionals. The skill mix of mental health teams therefore needs to be extended to include employment specialists and work-related welfare benefits. The employment specialists who provide the vocational services in mental health teams in South West London do not have mental health qualifications but instead they have experience and expertise in such areas as supported employment, JobCentre Plus, public relations, education and occupational psychology. And some also have the extremely valuable expertise born of personal experience of the challenges and possibilities of returning to work with mental health problems.

### Decide what you are going to stop doing

Sometimes attempts are made to change services by simply adding on extra programmes and leaving everything else as it was. This is not sufficient. A fundamental change in the guiding philosophy and purpose of services requires a more comprehensive review. We need to understand those elements of current services and professional roles that do not contribute to, or are actively antithetical to, changed services priorities and make difficult decisions about the way in which scarce resources are used. Care planning priorities and the resources devoted to day and sheltered work services may require particular scrutiny: could at least some of these be used to better facilitate access to open employment and other mainstream opportunities, as has been achieved in the United States?[15,16] In developing evidence-based supported employment services in South West London, a day centre and a hospital-based industrial therapy unit have been closed and another community sheltered work programme significantly downsized. The revenue released has been used to fund employment specialist posts within community mental health teams.

Similarly, it is not possible to ask already overstretched professionals to simply take on extra work. In South West London dedicated occupational therapy time has been earmarked for vocational work in community teams, in full recognition that this will limit other areas of their work. The maximum caseload of community teams has been reviewed in line with additional expectations (including assistance with vocational issues and work with carers) and mechanisms introduced to monitor and limit caseload size.

## Take a broader view of partnership working

It almost goes without saying that the development of employment opportunities must involve not only statutory health and social services providers but also the range of employment programmes that are provided in the voluntary sector. However, a range of non-mental health agencies are equally if not more central in enabling people to access employment: JobCentre Plus, Connexions, the economic development units of local authorities, chambers of commerce and major local employers (including health and social services) have a big part to play.

Links with organisations such as these are important not only to facilitate access for individuals with mental health problems but also as a route to securing extra funding for employment initiatives. Partnership bids which draw on the skills of different organisations are invariably more likely to be successful than those put in by a single agency to organisations like the Learning and Skills Councils and any of the European funding streams.

In South West London there has been great value in being a formal partner to bids, not only in enabling money to be secured for providing employment opportunities for people with mental health problems but also in directly strengthening other providers, especially those in the voluntary sector, to develop the skills to work more effectively with people with severe mental health problems. Partnership bids have been successful in securing funding from Europe and the Learning and Skills Council. A 'work preparation' contract with JobCentre Plus has also been won and income to employ additional staff has been furnished through a partnership of supported employment providers acting as a job broker under New Deal for Disabled People.

And we must not forget to look at our own backyard. Providers of health and social services are not simply providers of services, they are also major employers. Increasing access to employment must involve not only working with 'them out there', but also examining how we can increase access to employment within our own service.[10–13] The NHS is the largest employer in Europe. Together with local authorities and those contracted by health and local authorities to provide services, it comprises a huge section of the labour market. As the Secretary of State for Health has made clear:[18]

> A key objective of the Government is to enable all disabled people, including those with mental health problems, to make the most of their abilities at work and in the wider society and, as the largest public sector employer in the country, the NHS should also be making a significant contribution to delivering this agenda. The South West London Mental Health NHS Trust user employment project is an excellent example of such initiatives.

## Expect things to go wrong

Probably the biggest lesson that anyone attempting to change mental health systems must learn is that things will go wrong and it is all too easy for everyone to give up at the first sign of trouble to a chorus of 'I told you so'. We can minimise the impact of this by starting small, capitalising on the enthusiasm of a committed group of people who are determined to make it work and trying not to take risks that are too big to start with. But we cannot prevent setbacks. The key to system change is to be humble enough to pick up mistakes at the earliest possible point, open enough to learn from those mistakes and determined enough to make the necessary changes. Those who use our services are invariably our best teachers but we have to be prepared to heed what they say: what they have and have not found helpful, what else should be done or done differently.

However, it is important to remember that, in relation to employment, it is not only people with mental health problems themselves but also employers, other employment agencies, college tutors who are in receipt of our services. Again, we can learn as much from those who have chosen not to use our services, refused our approaches, turned down an applicant with mental health problems as from those who have availed themselves of our services.

There are many occasions when we reach the limits of our knowledge. If mental health services were really to restrict what they offer to those areas where there was a good evidence base, our activities would be significantly contracted. While it is critical that we look carefully at evidence concerning what works and continue developing this evidence base, the reality is that we are frequently forced to act on the 'best available evidence', which might be very slim indeed.

## Conclusion

We have drawn on our experience of trying to make employment central to mental health services in South West London to let readers of this book know how we have achieved what we have achieved and the lessons learnt along the way. We are still learning lessons, we hope we always will be, because the process of change is not one of grand restructuring in line with some well-established blueprint but one of organic growth, learning and development.

The challenge faced by anyone who experiences mental health problems is how to rebuild, or preferably maintain, a meaningful and satisfying life.[19-22] Work is central in that process and it must therefore be central to any mental health service.

## References

1 Chadwick P (1997) *Schizophrenia: the positive perspective. In search of dignity for schizophrenic people.* Routledge, London.
2 OPDM (2004) *Mental Health and Social Exclusion. Social Exclusion Unit Report.* Office of the Deputy Prime Minister, London.
3 Department of Health (1999) *National Service Framework for Mental Health – modern standards and service models.* Department of Health, London.
4 Becker D and Drake R (1993) *A Working Life. The Individual Placement and Support Program.* Dartmouth Psychiatric Research Center, New Hampshire.
5 Bond G, Drake, Meuser K *et al.* (1997) An update on supported employment for people with severe mental illness. *Psychiatric Services.* **48**: 335–45.
6 Bond G, Becker D, Drake R *et al.* (2001) Implementing supported employment as

evidence based practice. *Psychiatric Services.* **52**: 313–22.

7  Crowther R, Marshall M, Bond G *et al.* (2001) Helping people with severe mental illness to obtain work: systematic review. *British Medical Journal.* **322**: 204–8.

8  Bond G (2004) Supported employment: evidence for an evidence-based practice. *Journal of Psychiatric Rehabilitation.* **27**(4): 345–59.

9  Davis M and Rinaldi M (2004) Using an evidence-based approach to enable people with mental health problems to gain and retain employment, education and voluntary work. *British Journal of Occupational Therapy.* **67**(7): 319–22.

10  Perkins R, Buckfield R and Choy D (1997) Access to employment: a supported employment project to enable mental health service users to obtain jobs within mental health teams. *Journal of Mental Health.* **6**: 307–18.

11  Perkins R, Evenson E, Lucas S *et al.* (2001) What sort of 'support' in employment? *A Life in the Day.* **5**(1): 6–13.

12  Perkins R (1998) An act to follow? *A Life in the Day.* **2**: 15–20.

13  Perkins R and Selbie D (2003) Decreasing employment discrimination against people who have experienced mental health problems in a mental health Trust. In: A Crisp (ed.) *Every Family in the Land. Understanding prejudice and discrimination against people with mental illness.* Royal Society of Medicine Press, London.

14  Goddard K and Perkins R (2004) Making the most of those mountains of data: a case study in an adult mental health service. *Mental Health Review.* **9**(3):13–16.

15  Bailey E, Ricketts S, Becker D *et al.* (1998) Conversion of day treatment to supported employment: one year outcomes. *Psychiatric Rehabilitation Journal.* **22**(1): 24–9.

16  Becker D, Bond G, McCarthy D *et al.* (2001) Converting day treatment centers to supported employment programs in Rhode Island. *Psychiatric Services.* **52**: 351–7.

17  Perkins R (2002) Are your work colleagues one of 'them' or one of 'us'? *Open Mind.* **113**: 6.

18  Department of Health (2000) *The NHS Plan: a plan for investment, a plan for reform.* Department of Health, London.

19  Deegan P (1988) Recovery: the lived experience of rehabilitation. *Psychosocial Rehabilitation Journal.* **11**(4): 11–19.

20  Deegan P (1993) Recovering our sense of value after being labelled. *Journal of Psychosocial Nursing.* **31**(4): 7–11.

21  Anthony W (1993) Recovery from mental illness: the guiding vision of the mental health system in the 1990s. *Innovations and Research.* **2**(3): 17–24.

22  Repper J and Perkins R (2003) *Social Inclusion and Recovery. A model for mental health practice.* Bailliere Tindall, London.

# Index

T - #0670 - 101024 - C0 - 246/174/10 - PB - 9781857756678 - Gloss Lamination